The Artful Eater

The ARTFUL EATER

A Gourmet Investigates the Ingredients of Great Food

Second Edition, slightly revised
With a New List of Sources of Supply

Edward Behr

PUBLISHED BY
THE ART OF EATING
PEACHAM, VERMONT USA

Library of Congress Control Number 2004092171

ISBN 0-9747841-0-9 (pb.)

With photographs by the author

Design by Keith Chamberlin

The Art of Eating
PO Box 242
Peacham, Vermont 05862 USA

Acknowledgments

This book was written only through the generous help of many people who offered encouragement and freely shared their knowledge. Some debts are apparent from the text. Among the many more that are not, I thank Karen Hess for reading the manuscript in its entirety. And for reading particular chapters, I thank John Anderson, Ian Doré, John Hemingway, Hank Kaestner, Bill McAlpin, Gale McGranahan, Warrie Means, Robert A. Nitschke, Patrick Rance, and Roger Way. I am also grateful for the help of Ed Baum, Bob Becker, Jerry Bisson, Will Borgeson, Ron Buttery, Kay Caughren, Ken Coons, Keith Crotz, Marilyn Einhorn, Thom Feild, Harold Forde, Eric Germain, Lewis Hill, Ian Jackson, Philippe Jobin, Dennis Kauppila, Paul Kindstedt, John Labavitch, Jan Longone, Bill Luginbuhl, Harold McGee, Dwight Miller, Ted Myers, Ken Parr, Allen Stevens, Peter Stone, Frank Sugihara, George Trevelyan, Tom Vorbeck, Nach Waxman, and Judith Weber. Grace DiNapoli offered insights and helped in many ways. In addition, I have received much kind assistance from librarians, especially those of the Bailey/Howe Library of the University of Vermont, and John Barstow has given the book his patience and his conscientious editing. The careful copy editor of the revised edition was Nina Maynard.

On occasion in these pages, I may have failed to follow someone's good advice. Naturally I am the only one responsible for errors.

Contents

Preface to the Second Edition

Why revise and reprint this book? When it was first published by Atlantic Monthly Press in February 1992, sales were limited and it went quickly out of print. The eighteen chapters on ingredients became a sort of cult classic with their in-depth discussion of the way things taste. (The original working title of the book was *The Search for Flavor*.) I'll never write better about some of these foods; little that concerns their taste has changed.

I briefly considered updating the facts and stories, but that would have required delving into all the old research, investigating the new, and tracking down all the people whose stories I had told. The result would have been a new and probably awkward before-and-after book, and surely the voice of my early enthusiasm would have been lost. Instead, for this new edition I have lightly, carefully revised the text: simplifying, clarifying, focusing more on taste, correcting a few typographical errors and errors of fact. In particular, my telling of the earliest history of the cultivation of the tomato wasn't completely accurate, and I've relied on Sophie Coe's *America's First Cuisines* and Andrew Smith's *The Tomato in America* (though they don't agree in every detail) to correct it. The type in the original edition was small and cramped. Now, happily, the text has been entirely reset; Keith Chamberlin has given the book a handsome and more readable design.

Some comment on what has changed in the world of food in the last dozen years seems appropriate. The news on certain ingredients is discouraging. The environmental effects of salmon farming have become more controversial, and perhaps because international competition on price has affected methods, it appears to me that the taste of some farmed salmon has declined. I have gained more appreciation for the flavor of wild Pacific salmon. The situation of the wild Atlantic salmon, in both Europe and America, varies from tough in the southern part of its range to excellent in the far north, with further decline in the US and some uncertainty in Canada. A great disgrace is the deterioration in the quality of mass-produced pork and beef (most of the interest had already been taken from chicken). Some of what has been fed to pigs and cattle, including animal waste, is abominable not to say dangerous. Hogs are now raised to be so lean that the typical pork is dry and rubbery; nearly all comes from animals raised indoors under repulsive and inhumane conditions. Sadly, dry-cured Southern country ham is made almost exclusively from that mass-produced pork rather than from traditional, delicious fatty pork. Not only are beef cattle are raised using hormones, which are blamed for making the meat watery, but the animals are slaughtered younger than before, so they have a less beefy taste. (Chickens, which appear in this book as a source of eggs, continue to be raised indoors under cruel conditions. They are made to grow so fast that their meat tastes bland apart from, often, a vague, muddy off-flavor.)

I still don't like or buy supermarket apples. As for cream, an important subject of this book, superlative fresh cream remains scarce. Unfortunately, the dairy at Hill Farm has closed, but the Lazors of Butterworks Farm remain some of the best organic dairy farmers in the US. A few days ago I drove up to the farm to buy some of the raw cream, which was sweet, delicate — superb. (The best dairy news is that across the country many more good farm-made cheeses have come into existence, despite pressure from state and federal health inspectors who are not always well informed.) Among the suppliers that have disappeared is Tahitian Import/Export, a source of outstanding vanilla beans, and I don't know another on the same level. Starbucks, a novelty coffee roaster a dozen years ago, its stores just beginning to spread outward from Seattle, is now wholly mass-market and of no interest. Today there are so many outlets of so many coffee chains that there aren't enough excellent green coffee beans to supply even a fraction of them. Within this high-end "specialty" coffee market, nearly all the coffee is roasted very dark, so that the best qualities of the green beans — the ripe flavor of the coffee fruit coupled with fine acidity — have been almost eliminated. (But see the new list of suppliers at the end of the book.)

Other news is good. As I updated the suppliers' list, in the original categories I found a few I hadn't been aware of and some new ones, and I had no difficulty adding suppliers in a number of new categories. Certain further items have become available. For instance, I now know and appreciate *fleur de sel*, the whitest and purest form of unrefined sea salt, gathered from the surface of the salt pans, although for most uses I still prefer the stronger character of gray sea salt. (More recent study of the health effects of salt has been less supportive of my strong stand in favor of it, but I stick to my conclusion that for most people the use of salt to make food taste better is plain common sense.) Happily, a stream of delicious heirloom tomatoes has appeared, part of the huge increase in the amount of top-quality fresh produce grown across the country and sold especially at farmers' markets. Every seed catalog I know offers at least one or two old-fashioned, flavorful tomato varieties.

More small farms are producing decent and sometimes very delicious meats of many kinds, including well-marbled pork and beef, some from superior breeds outside the mainstream. For enabling a large number of family farms in the center of the country to raise pigs in the best old ways, Paul Willis of Iowa deserves enormous credit. He put together the network of farms that produces pork under the Niman Ranch label. (Across the US, individual small farms that wish to sell meat on their own are hampered not only by a lack of good small slaughterhouses but by a lack of skilled butchers to do the cutting.) In the last few years, an intelligent debate has arisen among chefs and farmers over the advantages of grass-fed as opposed to grain-fed cattle. My own opinion isn't yet formed, partly because there is so little well-marbled grass-fed beef to be had for making comparisons. (Some argue that leanness is part of the point of grass.) Fortunately, the taste of fat in general has become more fashionable, at least for now, though North Americans remain wary of fat in charcuterie, apart from bacon.

This book concerns cooking as well as eating. When I reread the original, I was surprised to find that here and there my cooking used to be more complicated than it is today. I would no longer think of putting orange liqueur in a custard. I was amazed to remember that I had written a recipe for "Salmon with Cream, Sauternes, and Raisins," whose layered richness now strikes me as caricature (as a matter of record I've left the recipe intact). In certain ways, my cooking has become more restrained and careful, reflecting my continued thought and greater experience. I no longer mix a portion of allspice with black pepper in a mill. And I find that as little as half a bay leaf is normally enough to flavor an entire braise. For almost all purposes, I've come to prefer classic *planifolia* vanilla to the more floral Tahitian species. But how many people are cooking at home in such a focused way?

In America, home cooking, as we all know, is done less and less by daily necessity and more and more as an occasional recreation. In general, in countries with modern economies, traditional regional cooking (which is more or less identical with home cooking) is in decline. Cooking has always evolved, whether on farms or in luxury restaurants, and the changes can be good, when they reflect a better quality of life: greater variety, higher-quality goods, less drudgery in the kitchen. But in recent decades so much change has occurred so quickly that the new elements, good and bad, aren't incorporated into the existing cooking. Instead they suddenly replace much of what made the old cooking valuable and distinct to begin with. And the same new elements are introduced around the world: we begin to eat all alike. Much of this new cooking is "creative." I remain discouraged by all but the best of that. As a rule it exploits powerful juxtapositions of foods or tastes for the sole reason of their unexpectedness, not for the sensual pleasure of the combinations, not for the way the foods complement or comment on each other.

I didn't in this book reveal — maybe I wasn't yet fully aware of — the extent to which the late Richard Olney, and especially his books *Simple French Food* and *The French Menu Cookbook*, have influenced me. Nor did I understand that all that is most interesting about food to me, as it was to him, concerns the five senses (plus the people one eats with, a separate story). The past attracts me only as it illuminates the present. I will always be grateful to Richard. One thing he recognized, which I overlooked before, was the importance of the "personality" of the cook. To quote from Olney's short preface to the revised edition (1985) of his classic *French Menu Cookbook*, "Food should be an expression of a cook's personality; a recipe executed by two individuals, in each of whom may reside a finely developed tactile sense, will produce, thanks to individual sensibilities, two different dishes, each of which may be flawless." (What Olney meant by "tactile sense," like what he meant by "simple food," is a subject in itself.)

When I wrote these essays, I lived, as I still do, in Vermont. I arrived here in 1973 as part of a wave of idealistic newcomers. I began to write about food in the mid-80s, when it was still possible to feel close to that back-to-the-land movement, though the flow of new arrivals had stopped. North Americans then retained a widespread interest in skilled handwork of all kinds, including farming and gardening. Today, we are more estranged than we were from traditional skills and rural life — from nature and the way food is produced. Yet very happily, because of the vogue for good food and the huge success and proliferation of farmers' markets, more Americans know and care about food. We've gained a new respect for one set of hand skills, those practiced by talented chefs. In the countryside in the last few years, more people have come from urban or suburban areas, often bringing with them capital and a romantic desire to produce food for sale, from meat and vegetables to cheese and bread. Some also bring a knowledge that makes them likely to succeed. Most of the earlier arrivals came without money — in those days land and living were cheap — and some in that generation are among our very best food producers. Others who have always lived in the countryside continue to make important contributions. All these producers share the belief that the best measure of quality in food is still the way things taste.

Preface to the First Edition

Five years ago, I began to write and publish a thin quarterly letter called *The Art of Eating*. I meant at first to give rudimentary instructions in eating well. I was somewhat ingenuous, yet I knew my real subject was not cooking but eating. I was answering for myself the basic questions: What is good food? And what makes it good? I've come to understand that there are very specific ways of posing these deceptively brief questions and that the answers are endless and complex. You never stop answering.

To my mind, the essence of good food is flavor — not health, certainly not speed of preparation or practicality. I have tried not to compromise in presenting what is aesthetically best. Knowing that, you can make the compromises you wish or must.

The phrase that I took for the title of my quarterly, "the art of eating," was probably inevitable, but I worried at the start that it was stolen from M.F.K. Fisher's famous collection of five books. In answer to my letter she wrote graciously, "Don't worry about thieving *The Art of Eating*. . . . I think I thieved it too, because it's taken from something said by Brillat-Savarin . . . something about how men and animals may eat and so on, but very few of them know the art of it." She invoked honor among thieves and signed herself "honorably yours."

Almost all the essays that appear in this book first appeared in the quarterly letter. They are appreciations of individual ingredients, the excellent raw materials on which all good food depends. They inspire both cook and eater: they teach. It is often said that no dish is better than its raw materials, but the implications may not be fully understood. Certain ingredients cannot be found without trouble. Some — immaculately fresh fruits and vegetables, vulnerable cheeses, aged meats, pastries, coffee beans roasted no more than a day before, well-crafted hard cider — are scarce or nonexistent in many parts of the US (certain cheeses cannot be had at all). As old bakers, sausage-makers, truck farmers, orchardists, even butchers and grocers have retired or passed away, much common knowledge of the past has been lost. The twentieth century has not been kind even to the memory of slow, careful artisanal ways, although a few of them are revived here and there. Our advanced knowledge is expressed in efficiency and mass-production. I have tried to discover and write some of the old truths about quality that are hardly known anymore.

Quality is primarily sensual and revealed in the way things taste, including, to some extent, their texture. Quality isn't conceptual or philosophical, as customers of health-food and gourmet stores sometimes seem to think. (There is an intellectual component to connoisseurship that involves bringing knowledge to the table, but this is largely memory of previous experiences together with knowledge and appreciation of the processes of production, and all of it is rooted in the senses.) Freshness in particular is an ephemeral goodness that disappears in a few hours or overnight. It certainly doesn't mean uncooked or not frozen. Refrigeration generally prolongs freshness — though it harms a few things — but it is no substitute for getting food as rapidly as possible from fields and woods and waters to the table. The only intervention should be that of a skilled artisan.

Is local food better? That depends. Yes — if it is produced well, though of course different regions are suited to different crops and animals, to different varieties and breeds and often species. In theory, local fruits and vegetables are fresher, picked riper, and grown from tastier, less invulnerable varieties than the ones that must withstand machine harvesting and long-distance shipping. Fruits for shipping long distances are picked underripe because softening is a large part of ripening, and soft fruit would be damaged in transit. Varieties to be grown for local sale can be chosen by the farmer primarily for exceptional flavor and texture. And if food is from your own locality, then you are more likely to be able to appraise and appreciate its quality. (Some experience at milking a cow, tending your own garden, and raising, killing, and dressing your meat contribute to the appraisal, although such experience isn't strictly necessary.) Also, local foodstuffs tend to be produced on a small scale by people who care more about quality and feel more accountable to their customers than do mass-producing strangers far away. Finally, buying local food helps to preserve local farms, a prerequisite for having local food.

I speak of local food rather than regional because "local" describes a smaller area, perhaps within a radius of a few miles. Assuming superior freshness, varieties, and care, the value of local food is that it contributes to a sense of place. Part of this is intangible: a kind of sentimental value simply in knowing that your meals come from nearby. But what is more important to a perceptive diner is that foods from different places taste different. And diversity in taste is probably the most interesting part of eating. Wildness is a part of the diversity; wild foods stimulate the senses in their own ways and provide untampered-with originals against which we can judge our achievements in domestication. Wine is the clearest and finest expression of local influence and is the model for other foods, but the flavor of almost every food worth eating expresses something of its geographic origins.

The source of local character is *terroir* — the French word, for lack of an English one. *Terroir* refers not only to the soil of a particular site but to the immediate climate, including rainfall, effects of elevation, exposure to wind and sun, influence of nearby bodies of water. There can also be an effect from nearby vegetation: a bordering forest of certain trees, a stand of wild berries. On the palate, the expression of *terroir* may be anywhere from imperceptible to dramatic.

A further layer of localism is added when a specific variety of plant or breed of animal is matched to *terroir*. As certain grapes best exploit the conditions of certain regions or vineyard sites, so milk from a region's traditional breed produces more characteristic cheeses. In France, breeds are legally specified for some controlled-place-name cheeses. And what is true for milk is true for meat. The union of land and plants and animals in a place often represents centuries of selection by farmers, herdsmen, gardeners, and nature.

In this book I only touch on the complexities of fermentation, although it strongly emphasizes local qualities. The ambient local microflora — strains of yeasts, bacteria, and molds — play a dominant role in traditionally produced wine, cheese, bread, aged sausage, vinegar, olives, and even some exceptional beers. Most often, these wild organisms are intentionally killed off by heat or sulfur and replaced by, or merely overwhelmed by, chosen laboratory strains that accomplish the fermentation or ripening. But some of the native wild organisms can produce marked differences in flavor. It is often difficult to separate the part of the taste they produce from the part resulting from the technique or the raw material. But given examples to compare, probably anyone could taste the differences among, for instance, British ales. For centuries British ale has been brewed using locally cultivated versions of the original wild yeasts, and in the only partly controlled microbiological climates of traditional British breweries, an array of wild organisms can exist alongside the cultivated ones. These wild organisms can contribute some complexity of flavor, as well as occasional off-flavors. Elsewhere, at least one kind of beer is still made by the ancient method of relying wholly on wild organisms. That beer is the highly distinctive Belgian *lambic*.

In the United States, examples of food or drink with strong regional or local ties are scarce. But one regional crop with venerable origins is the Narragansett Indian corn now selected for white color (a few plants still have red ears) and known as Rhode Island white flint. A few fields of it, only twenty or thirty acres in all, are still grown around Narragansett Bay, where the variety originated. A good part of the crop is stone-ground at Gray's Mill in Adamsville, on a spot where a succession of mills is believed to have operated continually since 1675. A competing mill on the other side of the bay is a mere hundred years old. Meal from Rhode Island white flint corn is still made into traditional Rhode Island jonnycakes, and the correct preparation of those is a subject of surprising interest and even controversy. Indigenous practices often enhance the uniqueness of local foods. Small decisions about technique may, for instance, determine the kind of wine, cheese, or bread that results, as they may determine the nature of a dish in the kitchen.

A specific accumulation of local influences cannot be reproduced anywhere else. Local production sets up a type against which to compare examples from different growers, different plots of ground, and different seasons. And foods that have arisen side by side over centuries tend to enhance one another, the obvious example being local drink with local bread and cheese. To appreciate local food, it helps to have some prior familiarity with the place as well as some knowledge of its food. Each evokes the qualities of the other. All this prolocalism is to say not that one shouldn't mix good products from everywhere, only that given the choice one ought to tip the balance toward the local.

It is important to understand the role of such variable raw materials in the kitchen. I've heard home cooks speak with annoyance of recipes that "don't work." And I'm sure some don't. But modern cooks often misunderstand the nature of a recipe. They tend to mistake it for the dish itself, although a recipe is a notation, an outline, a fluid thing. The dish takes its definite form only from the ingredients at hand and from the adjustments made by the cook, according to his or her skill and understanding. Scarcely any recipe can or should yield a fixed result. But the improvisation that goes on springs from ingredients, and the need for improvisation rarely if ever calls for the sort of inventiveness often referred to as "creativity." The dish itself is almost certainly a reiteration of a time-honored preparation. In the kitchen it's almost impossible to invent anything truly new.

Naturally, skill at cooking depends on skill at tasting. Most people know whether or not they have particular skills. They know that they are or aren't mechanics or dancers or mathematicians, but having mouths and stomachs, almost all believe they are skilled tasters-eaters. Yet taste, like other faculties, must be learned and developed through practice. And the most expert tasters in specific areas are often humble: to learn anything well is to discover over and over how little one knows.

I've never been able to give a satisfactory explanation of how I came to write about food, but I do know why I live where I do. I moved to the northeast corner of Vermont in the 1970s because it was a deeply rural place with a strong sense of a character apart. This character varied even with the terrain. The feeling in areas of tight wooded hills with few farms differed from that along the upper reaches of the Connecticut River valley, from that around the isolated and declining farming community of Norton next to the Canadian border, and especially from that in the more gentle open farming areas of Orleans County. Unfortunately, the distinctiveness of the entire region, like that of other places, is diminishing as the world becomes more homogeneous. But this is still a quiet, tolerant, protected place in which to live and work.

I write about very good food, the best, although that is a misleading word because there is rarely a single best. Rather there is a group of possibilities, often representing a rough consensus among connoisseurs. And to speak of only the best suggests disappointment, a striving for perfection that is seldom attained. No one can live for long at that pitch. Any cook makes concessions, choosing simplicity frequently or always. The important measures of the success of a meal are relaxation, stimulation, conversation — broad enjoyment. Work and calculation can go all the more awry because so much depends on serendipity — unforeseen unions of idiosyncratic raw materials, a conducive setting, and a receptive company in sympathy with the food, the cook, and each other.

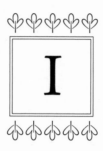

The Goodness of Salt

It's sad that the unclouded enjoyment of salt is a thing of the past. Salt is winning when a few grains of it are tasted in a tiny pinch, although that hardly begins to address the health campaign against this nutrient. Salt does raise blood pressure in the seventh or tenth of the population whose blood pressure is salt-sensitive. However, there is no evidence that people with normal blood pressure who avoid salt are reducing the chance of a future problem. The whole truth about salt is only beginning to be widely understood. Bureaucrats who issue alarmist guidelines see not individuals but an ill-informed mass of least common denominators, to be treated all alike. Ironically, until recently salt has been a metaphor for value, preservation, and permanence. Only during the 1980s did partial new knowledge turn the old symbol on its head. Now hardly anyone praises salt.

No passion like that for chocolate or champagne has ever declared itself for salt. Yet salt's potency in heightening the taste of food is unmatched and has been honored since ancient times. And salt has certain particular uses. It is imperative in bread dough to give a warm brown color to the baked crust. It conveniently lowers the freezing point of water in the salt and ice mix of old-fashioned ice-cream freezers — an application that has been exploited with increasing sophistication since the early vogue of fruit ices in the time of Catherine de Médicis. Salt enhances nearly every food, but its culinary significance is seen most clearly when it seasons breads, potatoes, and grains. Without it, they taste flat and almost metallic.

Without salt, there would be none of the delicious foods it preserves: ham, sausage, bacon, corned beef, smoked salmon, salt cod, anchovies, pickles, sauerkraut, cheeses, olives. Salting is often combined with two other fundamental means of preservation, drying and smoking, as in meats and fish. Before they are eaten, some salt-cured foods do have to be soaked for a day to rid them of enough salt to bring them back into the range of palatability, but the salt pungency of prosciutto that would be alarming in quantity merely sharpens the appetite in a small serving of thin slices over ripe melon or figs.

Nineteenth-century Americans ate more salt pork than they did fresh meat. The salty palate that resulted may explain the peculiar saltiness of American baked goods. The current generation of cookbooks has reduced the salt but until recently our pie pastry, Toll House cookies, sticky buns, banana bread, and other sweets have contained four times or more salt than their European equivalents. And the salt in our recipes is usually intensified by the alkaline taste of baking soda or powder and by the salt in salted butter. In the Old World, eggs and yeast are preferred leavenings to powders, and salted butter for baking is all but unheard of on the Continent. Even in Britain, unsalted butter was always used for the finest baking. The salty-sweet taste of our traditional baked goods is not so much good or bad as it is characteristic.

Salt has minor but worthy variety in type and flavor. Gray salt is the unrefined sea or bay salt, sometimes found in health-food and fancy-food shops, that looks dirty and has the stimulating flavor of the ocean. This salt has all the mingled salts of the sea and correspondingly less plain sodium chloride than refined salt. The French prefer a small sacrifice in flavor on behalf of delicate style: gray salt in the kitchen, white salt at the table, with occasional exceptions such as gray salt served with pot-au-feu.

Of the half-dozen kinds of salt currently on my shelf, gray Armorican salt made near the mouth of the Loire is the most interesting. Close behind are two kinds of coarse white crystals from Mediterranean France, as well as Maldon sea salt from Essex, England (from the Maldon Crystal Salt Company, the only remaining English maker of sea or bay salt). The usual refined white sea salt sold by health-food stores is more reasonably priced but has about half the desirable sea taste of the other four. A box of flaked kosher salt sat unused until it hardened and I threw it out. It was undistinguished and contained additives: contrary to the common impression, most brands of kosher salt do. Morton's plain salt for pickling (not iodized because iodine turns pickles black) also lacks interest, as does its table salt. Once I had some Hawaiian salt, and it was the most boring of all. I use the health-food store's refined sea salt for pasta water, the more expensive gray salt in most other cooking, and one or another imported salt on my table. It is a shame that for curing, where the kind of salt matters most, the cost of good gray salt is prohibitive.

Early in the twentieth century, when more scattered saltworks still survived, there was more variety to salt. The suffix -wich in an English place name — Norwich, Middlewich, Droitwich, Greenwich — means the site of a saltworks or brine spring. A native of the Kanawha River valley in West Virginia once wrote a book in which he lamented the passing of the Kanawha red salt that was no longer boiled from the brine springs in the town of Malden. It was colored by iron oxide, and its strong taste was prized for curing meat.

Salt deepens flavors and to an extent unites them, and it balances acidity and sweetness, helping to restore equilibrium when they are in excess. Salt plays not just against these basic tastes but against aromatic flavors, and it cuts the oily taste of fat. A vinaigrette for salad is a careful balance between oil and vinegar, a balance that turns on salt. That balance is famously difficult to achieve, easier with a prodigal use of oil, and the amount of salt is as often awry as that of the two liquids.

It is confusing that a set volume of salt weighs more or less depending on the variety. Coarse flaked salt weighs about half as much as a spoonful of granulated white salt, gray salt about two-thirds as much. Most recipes calculate for the granulated white, and any adjustments are up to the cook. A few otherwise knowledgeable cooks have the notion that sea salt is saltier than regular salt and that less is needed. To my palate, that just isn't so.

A salt grinder is sometimes used to grind coarse crystals "fresh" at the table, but I don't believe this freshness has any value. Rather, the appeal of grinding comes from the immediate lively effect of the fine salt particles and powder when they hit the tongue (the fineness depending on the grinder). Unfortunately, gray salt clumps and works poorly in either a grinder or shaker. It must be pinched.

Although the liking for salt is universal, each of us has a taste for a certain amount of it, based on what we are used to. And we often like more than we think we do. We clearly enjoy a good deal more than we need. For the cook, the correct amount of salt is no more than an average of individual tastes. Some professional cooks fail to recognize that their preferences are immoderate, so they don't reduce their salting to the average. Home cooks tend to underestimate the average, and they are often inconsistent. Or in the face of the campaign against salt, they don't salt at all. They may not realize that part of the pleasure they take in a meal at a good restaurant comes from well-salted — skillfully salted — food.

A salt grinder, shaker, or dish should always be on the table so that individuals can season food to taste, especially such foods as roasts, which don't come fully salted from the kitchen. I respect and sympathize with those who have to restrict their use of salt, but some zealous puritans would like everyone to cut down on salt because a small percentage would benefit from abstinence. These fearful proselytizers have no spirit, no *joie de vivre*. Does the sensual, the aesthetic, have no value in life? To those with high blood pressure it may be an injustice on the part of Fate, but it is impossible to enjoy food fully without salt. Salt is part of the structure of taste. Its use isn't a weakness, but an intelligent application of the senses.

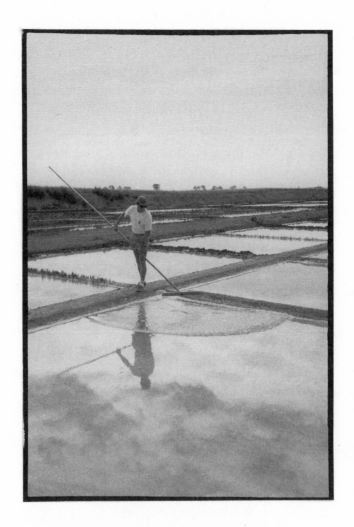

*Gathering salt from centuries-old
carreaux off the Atlantic coast of France.
Ile de Ré, 1996.*

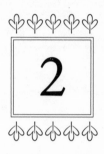

2

A Ripe,
Flavorful Tomato

The tomato is a South American native, and even today the greatest concentration of wild tomatoes is found in the coastal mountains of Ecuador and Peru, the area of its ancient origin, and not far away on the Galápagos Islands. Not long after Cortés conquered the Aztecs in Mexico, the first tomatoes were carried back to Europe. Tomatoes, when the Europeans arrived in the New World, were being cultivated in Central America, but curiously, there is no archaeological or other evidence that they were being or had been cultivated anywhere else. From early descriptions, it appears those cultivated tomatoes may have existed in colors from yellow through deepest red to pink. There may have been smooth, smallish globes; large, flattened shapes with irregular lobes and ribs; elongated ovals; and some fruit with nipple-shaped tips. All this is uncertain because European observers weren't always clear when they wrote and didn't always know what fruit they were looking at. Our word tomato comes from the Aztec *tomatl*, which means "plump fruit" (according to the anthropologist Sophie Coe) and embraces not only tomatoes but similar-looking fruit, such as the tomatillo; the tomato was specifically the *xitomatl*. In the United States, some confusion about species lasted even into the mid-nineteenth century.

The earliest record of the tomato in Europe is the description in

1544 by the Renaissance botanist Pier Andrea Mattioli of Siena. Ten years later, he recorded the common Italian name for them, giving the plural *pomi d'oro* (not far from Italian *pomodori* today), so presumably he had a yellow variety. By 1560 tomatoes are believed to have been grown in Italy for cooking, and there is evidence that the Spanish were cooking with them by a similar date. Tomatoes were not so readily received into kitchens in France, where in 1586 they were called *pommes d'amour*, from the earlier, mistaken idea, adhered to by Mattioli, that they were related to the mandrake, one of whose names was "love apple." (In Spanish and Portuguese, *tomates* and *tomatas* held sway; names were not entirely settled for 250 years.) The early-seventeenth-century herbalists Gerard and Parkinson indicate that tomatoes were then grown in England but not yet eaten. (According to *The Country Farm*, 1606: "The fruit being eaten it provoketh loathing and vomiting.") The period of hesitation lasted four centuries in some places.

The first tomato plants brought to Europe bore fruit that was large and irregular, and the colors were both red and yellow. The large, irregular tomato was the type that arrived in North America, perhaps in the mid-eighteenth century, and probably from Spain or Italy. A second major type — smaller and smooth — had been recorded in 1700 in Paris; it arrived in the United States later than the large red. This, called the love apple in America as in France, was grown primarily for its appearance. The name fell out of use the more the tomato was eaten.

Thomas Jefferson, the most famous early North American gardener, listed "tomatas" among vegetables grown in Virginia gardens in the early 1780s. Probably he meant the gardens of the wealthy, and it is unclear how frequently they ate the fruit. Tomatoes don't appear in his records of his own garden until 1809; he grew and served a Spanish and a dwarf variety. The history of the early use of the tomato is sometimes disputed, but it seems fairly certain to me that the well-to-do were the avant-garde in tomato consumption for half a century or more.

The popular embrace of the tomato was described by Robert Buist, nurseryman and seedsman, in *The Family Kitchen Gardener*, published in 1847:

> In 1828–9 it was almost detested; in ten years more every variety of pill and panacea was "extract of Tomato." It now occupies as great a surface of ground as cabbage, and is cultivated the length and breadth of the country. As a culinary dish it is on every table from July to October.

Sixteen years later, Fearing Burr, Jr., wrote in *The Field and Garden Vegetables of America*:

> In this country, its cultivation and use may be said to have increased fourfold within the last twenty years; and it is now so universally relished, that it is furnished to the table, in one form or another, through every season of the year. To a majority of tastes, its flavor is not at first particularly agreeable; but by those accustomed to its use, it is esteemed one of the best . . . of all garden vegetables.

As the tomato increased in popularity, the number of varieties offered by seedsmen increased from one or two (a large and a small) to four or more. By the 1850s there were red and yellow large ribbed tomatoes, smooth red and yellow love apples, red and yellow pear shapes, and more. Then very quickly there followed a multitude of varieties with more specific names, such as Lester's Perfected, Fejee, and The Cook's Favorite. Late in the century the most popular varieties included Acme, Hathaway's Excelsior, and General Grant, all of them since disappeared. By then, tomatoes were being shipped green from Florida and Bermuda to supply the northern demand out of season. And if only one vegetable was grown in the family garden, it was the tomato.

In the hands of nineteenth-century breeders, not only did varieties proliferate but tomatoes themselves changed. U.P. Hedrick, prolific recorder of American agriculture, wrote in *A History of Horticulture in America* (1950):

> A landmark in the breeding of tomatoes was the introduction of the Trophy, a little after the middle of the century. It was a product of Dr. Hand, Baltimore County, Maryland, who began breeding tomatoes about 1850. In his work he crossed the small, smooth love-apple, commonly grown in gardens as an ornamental, with the several larger garden varieties then being grown. These garden tomatoes all bore much convoluted fruit with the skin running deeply in the convolutions. The Trophy was a solid mass of flesh and juice, with small seeds, and the smooth skin of the love-apple. Trophy long remained a standard sort, and became the parent of the several races and hundreds of varieties we now grow.

But Trophy itself is said to have "run out" by 1900.

The frenzy of breeding that followed the Civil War produced countless varieties. Rather than being intentional crosses, or hybrids, they were often selected from a single outstanding plant in a field, from whose seed plants and more seed were propagated. In succeeding years, the grower had to continue to preserve the seed of only the most characteristic plants, or the so-called variety would degenerate to some uncertain ancestor. Even well-maintained varieties were very mixed in heredity. The problem was still serious enough in 1933 that a top USDA horticulturalist wrote a booklet describing in detail the proper characteristics of the major commercial varieties, in the hope that commercial seed could be made more true to type.

Some of the old varieties were genuine improvements. The large rough fruits were made to ripen earlier, grow meatier, and certainly they were made smooth. Yield was increased, and varieties became regionally adapted through selection by gardeners and by nature.

The wave of plant breeding didn't stop. A 1910 gardening manual advised: "Varieties pass out and new ones come into notice, so that a list is of small permanent value." The breeders were now putting most of their efforts into developing disease resistance. The *Yearbook of the United States Department of Agriculture, 1937* listed attributes of recently developed varieties, but tellingly it made only one reference to taste; Rutgers was said to have "flavor for juice." And with few exceptions, the varieties introduced in the last half of the century have been chosen for characteristics other than good flavor. Looking back at the whole history of the tomato, there seems no reason to believe that the best pre-Columbian tomatoes weren't as delicious as the best of today's.

The taste of the tomato, like that of other fruits (botanically the tomato is a berry), is built on a structure of sugars, primarily fructose and glucose, and acids, primarily citric, but also malic and minor quantities of others. The sugars are distributed throughout the tomato, but there is about twice as much acid in the gel surrounding the seeds as there is in the flesh. Sweet and sour we perceive on the tongue, but the most characteristic part of tomato flavor is, of course, aromatic, perceived in a complex interaction between nose and mouth.

Taste is highly subjective, but nevertheless you can scrutinize its components. At the USDA's Western Regional Research Center in Albany, California, Dr. Ronald Buttery and a small group are investigating the aromatic compounds that contribute to tomato flavor. Working with a number of different varieties, they have found two to four times as much of these volatile compounds in the flesh as in the translucent gel (with a small extra dose next to the skin). While many more flavor components have been identified, Dr. Buttery's laboratory is looking at about thirty-five compounds that appear in significant quantities, about ten of which contribute to flavor, the rest being below the threshold of human perception.

The main component of fresh tomato flavor has the unsentimental name of (Z)-3-hexenal. This and other aromatic compounds are formed only when the fruit is sliced or chewed (the same being true of some of the flavors in melons, apples, and certain other fruits). But the compound is highly unstable; if a plate of sliced tomatoes sits for twenty minutes, about half of the substance disappears. (Salting slows the loss.) The flavor constituents of cooked or canned tomatoes are largely different; no (Z)-3-hexenal remains. And part of the canned-tomato taste results from interaction with the metal can. Most people are said to like this taint, but purists put up their own fruit in glass jars.

There is something almost unkind about having the basic, gratifying smell of a tomato quantified and labeled, but the definition is not so absolute. Dr. Buttery says there is not a single tomato flavor but many shades of flavor, citing differences among red, orange, and yellow types. Researchers are looking for commercial strains that don't lose their flavor in the chill of refrigeration (an issue with tomatoes), and Dr. Buttery thinks a perfectly delicious supermarket tomato is fully probable. At the University of Massachusetts experiment station in Waltham, Dr. Clark Nicklow has been guided by his own palate in developing exceptionally flavorful tomatoes adapted to the Northeast — and specifically for commercial growers. They have begun to appear in supermarkets, and he hopes they will displace the tomatoes shipped in from farther south. He has been working with tomatoes since 1958: "I probably taste a couple of thousand tomatoes each summer." Dr. Nicklow looks for taste, yield, and disease resistance, but success with consumers will come only from superior taste, which he is confident he has achieved in experimental varieties. In the past, his hybrids have won first and second place in both the commercial and home-garden categories in the annual best-tasting tomato contest run by the Massachusetts agriculture department. (He supplements these main choices with strains that are more acid or more sweet to please consumers who prefer those types.)

Two more things are indispensable to a flavorful tomato, besides variety and the way it is grown: it must ripen completely on the vine, and once picked it must remain warmer than 55 degrees Fahrenheit. The earlier a tomato is picked before full ripeness, the less flavor it will have; the more time it spends below 55 degrees, the less flavor it will have. Warmth is essential to aroma. Tomatoes should never be refrigerated.

The notorious hard supermarket tomato has been improved, but it still comes from one or another inferior variety, and even then it has been picked green or half-ripe to withstand the rigors of shipping and to give it a long shelf life. Often such a tomato is artificially "ripened" in a benign atmosphere of ethylene gas. The term "ripen" as used by big growers is generally a euphemism for redden, which is not at all the same thing. With few exceptions, the hothouse tomatoes sold in supermarkets are hardly better than these "gas tomatoes."

Many people have fond memories of old crops, but Dr. Henry Munger, professor emeritus and highly respected plant breeder at Cornell University, is a strong advocate of what has been accomplished in recent years, and he cares about flavor. He says, "We forget how much crops have improved. Recollections get distorted by time. People just don't realize how much better things are today than they were before." He recounts a story of people who kept telling the owner of a farm stand how good the old Golden Bantam corn used to be. Finally, the farmer grew it, and the people bought it once, ate it, didn't like it, and never bought it again. Dr. Munger is not patient with romanticism about the vegetables of the past ("It annoys me no end"), but he concedes that those flavorful tomatoes that were developed by breeders in past decades weren't accepted for commercial introduction. He grew the old John Baer tomato when he was a boy and liked its flavor, but the variety had bad problems with cracking.

Typically, the fruit of a flavorful tomato variety ripens in mid- to late season, and the vines are indeterminate (they grow to ten feet or more, never stopping until they are killed by frost). Dr. Munger has shown in breeding experiments that an indeterminate vine produces 20 to 25 percent more sugars than a determinate vine of the same variety. The reason is that the indeterminate plant has more leaves per cluster of fruit. The extra foliage more fully exploits the sun: more photosynthesis occurs. And more photosynthesis in the leaves results in more sugars and other solids and aromatics accumulating in the fruit. The ideal growing environment contains a balance of nutrients, water, and light. In regions where wilts and other diseases are serious problems, it may be an essential gardening tactic to plant a resistant variety that will retain its foliage and so develop its full flavor.

Just how good are the older varieties (many still with irregular lobed fruit) compared to the new ones? The quality of the specific strain of the old variety is important. Any variety responds somewhat differently under different growing conditions. Most backyard gardeners have tried only a few different tomatoes, maybe not the best new ones. Since as a rule new varieties are healthier and more prolific, home gardeners' sticking with the familiar might account for the durable sales of some old varieties. However, except for Henry Munger's mixed reactions, all the reports that I've heard from gardeners, seed companies, and garden writers indicate that the best-tasting old varieties are at least as delicious as the best-tasting new ones — a few perhaps more so. And a higher percentage of the surviving old varieties taste exceptionally good. (One caution in tasting to compare flavor: the blossom end of a tomato is invariably superior to the stem end, as is the case with melons, peaches, citrus, and some other fruits.)

Two older American varieties that are often standards of comparison for flavor are Ponderosa, a pink (actually, pinks have red flesh and translucent unpigmented skin; the color is more of a washed-out red), and the famous Beefsteak. This, also known as Red Ponderosa, dates from around 1900. The tomato usually mentioned by the network of seed-saving gardeners as being the most flavorful of all is the red-pink Brandywine, said to be an Amish variety from 1885 or earlier. It is now available from such seed companies as Southern Exposure Seed Exchange and Pinetree Garden Seeds. Many of the best-liked older varieties have meaty fruits with little acidic gel and therefore few seeds, but still enough acid to show off their sugar. (A few years ago one midwestern seed catalog claimed nonsensically that its best-tasting tomato was "free of acidity," which no tomato is.) Sweet flesh pleases some people, but others associate intense tomato flavor with greater acidity. The pink and orange tomatoes are perceived as less acidic, though generally they have the usual level of acid, only it is masked by a higher than usual sugar content. Those who aren't familiar with the pink and orange are often wowed by their flavor; others find them simply mild.

There are many other flavorful varieties to select out of the great wash of insipid ones. Some are: Abraham Lincoln (1923), Big Boy (1949), Bonny Best (considered the same as John Baer, 1908), Carmello (a modern French hybrid), Delicious (1964), Dona (another more recent French hybrid), Jubilee (1943, orange), Mandarin Cross (a recent Japanese hybrid), Oxheart (offshoot of Ponderosa, 1925, pink), Pearson (1936), Persimmon (a persimmon-colored heirloom said to come from Mexico), Pruden's Purple (a purplish pink heirloom), Super Marmande (an improved version of the old French Marmande), Supersteak (1980), and Tappy's Finest (a family heirloom from 1948, pink-red). Of all these, only the acidic Pearson has determinate vines, and maybe it doesn't belong on the list.

Unhappily, disease often besets the old varieties, although even when the foliage is harmed they generally continue to bear fruit. And it may be that during the last century and a half, the diseases themselves have evolved and worsened under the conditions of monoculture. In humid climates, a home gardener can keep the plants well separated and staked or trellised to allow better air circulation, which helps keep the leaves dry and healthy. Where I live in northern Vermont, the brief summer is always hot and humid for spells, and the tomatoes suffer. Having experimented with pruning to one or two long branches as well as with allowing the vines to grow at will, I now suspect that whenever foliage is pruned, the flavor of the fruit suffers. In particular, it seems to be a mistake to follow the often-advised practice of pinching out the "suckers" that sprout in every angle where a side branch leaves a main stalk. It's much less work to grow unpruned plants in tall, broad-meshed wire cages and simply push errant branches back through the mesh. In most outdoor commercial growing, no training at all is required, and disease-resistant varieties are allowed to sprawl over the ground on plastic.

One of the great difficulties in obtaining flavorful tomatoes outdoors in a temperate climate is rain. Any but the lightest rain inflates the fruit with water, diluting its flavor and frequently cracking the skin. Certain varieties are especially prone to cracking. I have planned a small tomato greenhouse for my garden in the hope that warm plants, dry foliage, and relatively dry soil will justify the effort. A much easier solution is to slope the ground away from tomato plants and cover the soil with plastic, so water will run off. In the model tomato climate of Sicily, after the moist spring, dry culture is traditionally practiced during the sunny, hot, rainless summer; the bloated irrigated crops are disdained for local use. Tomatoes grown in Israel have been irrigated with saline water in order to produce more concentrated flavor. In a temperate climate, gardeners can only hope that rain won't hit just before the harvest of high-season fruit.

The very best tomatoes of all are grown under conditions of low moisture in soil that is only moderately enriched. Plenty of humus from natural compost, with no concentrated forms of fertilizer, may help flavor. Certainly lime enhances flavor and probably so does adding a range of trace minerals in the form of ground rock powders, including rock phosphate and greensand. Overall, a degree of stress on the plants — from low moisture, high heat, and only a moderate supply of nutrients — appears to intensify flavor.

I have grown only a few superlative tomatoes in northern Vermont. None of the touted, recently introduced early bearing varieties, wherever they are grown, has enough time to develop flavor before the fruit ripens. Raising them isn't worthwhile. Gardeners in cool areas should set out large, stocky plants — plants that are wider than they are tall and that have buds but not flowers. Plants can be permanently affected by cold weather during this early period, and they should as necessary be protected under plastic at night or grown for a period under spun-bonded polyester fabric, which breathes and allows water to pass through. Black plastic mulch under the plants, however unecological and unaesthetic, helps to heat the soil. If the first small fruits set on the vine are chilled below about 45 degrees Fahrenheit, they never develop good flavor. At the end of the season, new blossoms and tiny fruit should be cut off so as to direct the plant's energy toward the remaining large fruit.

I have often thought, during that impressively brief moment when the tomatoes in my northern garden could not be better, that I could eat a salad of such tomatoes every day of the year. Probably anyone could. Nothing from the garden tastes so essential. The acid-tinged sweet richness is like summer distilled on a plate. Bare slices with perhaps the contrast of coarse salt on the surface play to the unadulterated flavor. To justify dressing them with a vinaigrette, you must have very good red-wine vinegar. Tomato flavor is attractively complicated by the peppery-anise taste of basil, the herb with the greatest affinity for tomatoes (followed by the smoother flavor of tarragon). For sauce, especially one that is to simmer a long time, a somewhat acidic tomato at the start will retain the needed slight edge of acid piquancy to the end, balancing the concentration of sugar and tomatoeyness. The San Marzano variety, originally from the town of San Marzano sul Sarno between Pompeii and Salerno, generally fills the need, even when canned and imported. To avoid a mistake, look for the "San Marzano" on the can and see that neither sugar nor salt is listed as an ingredient.

The very best tomatoes ripen at the height of the season. They spend more time on the plant and accumulate more flavor during the summer's heat without yet being diminished by the cool fall. If all the desirable forces of moisture, nutrients, and care coincide, the fruit is sweeter and more intensely aromatic than the usual North American garden tomato. A gardener in a dry climate can achieve the ideal, and perfectionists elsewhere may try sheltering vines in a greenhouse. But even outdoor temperate-climate gardeners can take satisfaction in luscious, delicious, and — barring rain — concentrated fruit.

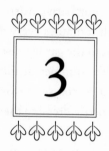

3

Labiatae: Some Herbs
of the Mint Family

The Labiatae, the members of the mint family, include, besides mint, a number of herbs that are fundamental to Western cooking: thyme, marjoram, oregano, basil, sage, rosemary, and savory. Also in the family are ancient herbs with lesser culinary value, such as lavender, hyssop, lemon thyme, horehound, betony, catnip, lemon balm, bergamot (bee balm), germander, pennyroyal, and dittany of Crete. Most of the thirty-five hundred members of the mint family are no bigger than our garden herbs, though some are larger shrubs and a few are vines or trees. In nature, these species are centered on the Mediterranean basin, but according to wildflower books, about 135 are native to or naturalized in the northeastern quarter of the United States and in southeastern Canada.

The labiates are named for the liplike opening of their flowers (*labium* being Latin for "lip"), though the lips are scarcely distinguishable in the simple flowers of most of the herbs. Aside from the clearly lipped flowers of sage, a protruding lower petal, more tongue than lip, is usually the only clue that a flower belongs to the mint family. (Confusingly, the Labiatae have an alternative name — the Lamiaceae, after the lamiums, or dead nettles, whose features make them more or less a model for the family.) Other characteristics are an aromatic scent, square stems, simple leaves in opposite pairs, and, among labiate herbs, a flower color between blue and purple.

Exceptions are the red flowers of bergamot and pineapple sage (which does have a pineapple scent but is of little use in the kitchen). In some of the wild herbs, the flowers appear in a range of colors from white to blue to purple, and in cultivars encouraged by gardeners, those colors are augmented by a definite pink. The flowers of the culinary herbs usually rise above the foliage on stems, mounting in distinct pairs in either whorls or a dense column.

The source of each herb's aroma is the oil in glands located on leaves, stems, and blossoms. Looking closely, you can almost see the glands, especially on the smooth leaves of basil; they are scattered among (and are actually larger than) the visible pores on both sides of each leaf. The blossoms often have better flavor than the leaves do, as you discover by tasting. Most blossoms are easily separated from the picked stems by rubbing backwards, although a sage flower must be plucked from the tough calyx that holds it.

Spearmint, peppermint, apple mint, and the thirty or more other mints — a confusion of species — belong to the genus *Mentha*. Menthe was a water nymph and mistress of the god Hades, and like water nymphs, wild mints are found next to streams. In North America, they are escapes from the mint planted by the earliest European settlers. Most of the wild mints divide by scent into two camps, one more or less spearmint and the other clearly peppermint (usually with a purple-black stem). In the garden, mints must be confined in a pot or banished to a far corner where the aggressive spreading of their runners will do no harm. I seldom cook with mint and I grow only one, an apple mint that a friend brought from Maine. Apple mint has the flavor of spearmint, which is much more useful than peppermint. Mint deserves more use than I give it. A pizza I once topped with oil-stewed onions and herbs, mostly mint, was approved by the eaters, who didn't guess the herb.

The major labiate herbs have been written about so often that here I have taken more note of some less well-known ones. But it is worth mentioning that the dried whole branches of wild oregano blossoms imported from Greece are greatly superior to any other form of oregano, fresh or dried. Also, the strong, direct taste of winter savory, a perennial, seems preferable to the weaker, vaguer one of summer savory, an annual.

The first year I planted hyssop, it became a favorite. The crushed leaves have an attractive perfume, something like a resinous combination of savory and thyme. Once upon a time, hyssop was present in nearly every garden; it was probably as common as an onion. Some of the earliest garden writers took it so much for granted that they didn't trouble to mention it. Hyssop may have been looked down on as pottage for the poor. It is easy to grow, even in poor soil, though it prefers lime and a well-drained spot in the sun. The herb is winter hardy, little bothered by insects, loved by bees, and blooms over a relatively long period with erect stalks of blue flowers. For centuries hyssop was a potherb, an ancient use that, as near as I can tell, persisted in the United States into the nineteenth century. And it has long been used in salads. In my garden I enjoy the vigorous, round weedy shape that hyssop assumes on its own, but Elizabethan and Tudor gardeners clipped it into miniature hedges for knot gardens.

The modern neglect of the herb on both sides of the Atlantic results from its moderate bitterness, which becomes strong during a drought. With careful use (chopped in salad or briefly cooked in sauce with other herbs), hyssop's perfume is reinforced and no bitterness is apparent. The taste is not clear like mint's but muddy, complex, evocative. In the secret recipe for Chartreuse, with its innumerable herbs and spices, hyssop is supposed to be a leading ingredient together with lemon balm, angelica, cinnamon, mace, and saffron, according to the *Larousse gastronomique*. As in other old-fashioned herbal liqueurs, many of the herbs were intended to be medicinal.

Anise hyssop is neither anise nor hyssop but belongs to a separate genus in the mint family. (Anise belongs to the parsley family.) Anise hyssop is a tender perennial that eagerly self-sows in my climate; it has a marked licorice taste and some of the most prominent, long-lasting flowers of any herb. By early September, mine is thirty inches high and covered with three-inch-tall clusters of bright purple flowers, most of them actually colored calyxes whose petals have long since fallen. Anise hyssop goes into salads and may once have had other uses.

The lavender in my garden is Munstead Dwarf, named after the home of the English garden designer and writer Gertrude Jekyll, who grew this cultivar. In her books, Miss Jekyll doesn't mention lavender as being in her kitchen garden, so she must have grown it purely for its scent and appearance. Several British writers early in the twentieth century asserted the superiority of lavender raised commercially in Britain over the better-known lavender raised in France. A number of types do exist, and climate or cultural methods may have made a difference. The flavor of lavender and other herbs is improved by adding lime to the soil, emulating the limestone soil around the Mediterranean. But lavender was not traditionally a culinary herb, at least not in Provence, where now it forms part of the standard mixture of Provençal herbs sold to tourists to take home and cook with.

Of the culinary labiates, only basil and summer savory are annuals, easily raised from seed. The perennials can be raised from seed, but thyme, winter savory, rosemary, and mint are slow or reluctant to germinate. They are best acquired as plants. And unlike buying seed, you can smell and taste a plant before buying it and be sure of an excellent aroma. Later the plants can be increased by division, by rooting cuttings (in damp sand), or by layering (burying side branches and separating them from the parent after they take root). Rosemary and the best-flavored marjoram are tender perennials, but the other major perennials are hardy. Over the years, the herb garden tends to become a collection of particularly well flavored and interesting varieties.

An herb garden often seems like a bee garden. Bees have their preferences in flowers. They ignore red ones because they don't perceive red, and they are especially attracted to the blues and purples of the Labiatae. Concentrating on collecting nectar, bees are little likely to sting — sympathetic companions for the gardener at work.

Herbs are some of the easiest of plants to appreciate, yet it adds to one's pleasure to place them in the context of whole families. Knowing which herbs are related, you begin to study the less celebrated kin more closely. And, once familiar with the family in the garden, you recognize members in the wild and understand nature more as a whole.

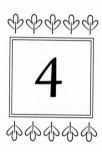

4

A Mussel Primer

The ordinary blue mussel, long known and ignored on American coasts, is the one beloved in France and Belgium, perhaps the greatest mussel-eating countries in the world. *Mytilus edulis* inhabits the band of shore that lies between the tides, although it can be found far below the low-tide mark. In Europe the supply of wild mussels cannot satisfy demand, and so most European mussels are farmed, primarily in Spain and also in France, Belgium, the Netherlands, and elsewhere. And lately in North America, mussels have been farmed in increasing numbers in response to an awakening market, although here most commercial mussels are still wild ones. They are found commonly along the Atlantic coast from the Arctic to North Carolina, and along the Pacific coast from southeastern Alaska to northern Baja California. In the lower portion of the rich intertidal strip, the mussel dominates such competitors as rockweed and barnacles, especially in areas exposed to surf. A few creatures, including starfish, the dogwhelk, and the green crab, regard the mussel as food. The mussel itself, like a number of other marine animals, feeds by filtering water for plankton and miscellaneous organic debris.

The mussel fastens itself to rocks, to other mussels, or to whatever support is available by means of the greenish beard that protrudes from its shell. The beard is properly known as the byssus, and its threads are very strong. If you are cleaning mussels, you will find that while you can pull the byssus free, the threads of the byssus are themselves nearly impossible to break. The gluelike threads are extruded one at a time from a gland at the base of the dark foot (the same as the neck of a clam), and the mussel sticks them onto adjacent objects. The strands harden on contact with seawater and harden faster in rougher water. A mussel, especially a young one, does not necessarily remain anchored in place. If it requires a better location for feeding or is broken loose by surf, it will release its beard and move with water currents and help from its small foot, searching for a more hospitable anchorage to again make itself fast.

On coasts where they are ignored by people living nearby, mussels are often plentiful and easy to gather at low tide. But before you do that, it is essential to know that there is no pollution from chemicals or sewage. And to know that mussel harvesting hasn't been banned because of the toxic luminescent organisms that produce red tides — dinoflagellates of the genus *Gonyaulax*. When they bloom in the water, they make shellfish extremely poisonous. (In great concentrations, these tiny organisms do color the water red.) Although harmful to humans, the dinoflagellates do little harm to the shellfish themselves, which take them in as part of their filter feeding. The problems of water quality and health are closely monitored by government authorities, since there is considerable economic interest in shellfish.

A second mussel of some importance in North America is the California mussel (*M. californianus*), which with its somewhat more rugged byssus lives in the Pacific surf, while the blue mussel is found in bays and quieter Pacific waters. The shape of either mussel's shell helps it to withstand the force of breaking waves. The California mussel is considered by some people to have a slightly less subtle and attractive flavor, but in the kitchen the blue mussel and the Mediterranean mussel (*M. galloprovincialis*) are the same. Frequently for sale on the West Coast, and well regarded, is the main culinary mussel of Asia, the green-shelled *Perna canaliculus*, or New Zealand mussel as it is usually called here. And there are less-common edible mussels, such as the Mediterranean date-shell mussel.

North American mussel farming began in about 1980, and in this context the word *farmed* carries a range of meanings. No one in the United States claims to sell wild mussels, but some "farmed" mussels are no more than cleaned-up wild ones. In France, the long-standing cultural practice is to suspend the mussels off the sea bottom on *bouchots*, wooden stakes, which is convenient for workers and keeps the mussels clean but exposes them regularly at low tide. (Mussels may have been farmed since classical times. France's claim to being the home of mussel aquaculture is based on the story of a thirteenth-century Irishman who, shipwrecked on the French shore, is supposed to have originated the *bouchot* technique and then gone into the mussel business.) Spanish production is concentrated on the Galician coast, where the preferred method is to suspend the mussels on ropes in water deep enough that they are continuously immersed and feeding. This method produces the fastest, tenderest, plumpest results.

Most American farmed mussels are kept continuously submerged for the same reason: a slow-growing mussel makes chewy eating. Farmed mussels typically reach market size of two to three inches in six months to three years, while wild mussels take five to seven years to reach the same size. In nature, the mussels highest up the shore are the slowest growing of all (cold water also slows growth), and, like other intertidal mussels, they are tough from resisting the pull of waves. The natural beds in the intertidal zones are often overcrowded, with as many as two thousand seed mussels per square foot; individual female mussels produce millions of minuscule eggs, so small as to be distributed like plankton with the currents. Most US farmed mussels are raised on carefully chosen and manicured sections of the bottom. These beds are seeded with about half-inch mussels at roughly twenty per square foot. On the West Coast, cultured mussels are hung in bags on racks to keep them off the bottom and away from predators. Scarcely any US mussels are rope farmed.

Those who take care in raising mussels say theirs are not only tenderer and plumper but also sweeter and tastier than wild ones. The question of flavor is a little more complicated than that, and the distinction between a wild and a farmed mussel can be artificial. Rather than being fed a specially devised diet, cultured mussels eat the same waterborne plankton and miscellany as wild ones. And like bottom-cultured mussels, some wild mussels occur naturally in deeper water below the low-tide mark. These are the fastest growing and tenderest of the wild. Some people find good wild mussels to taste better than the very quickly grown cultured ones. The definite variety in mussel flavor reflects place and time of year — primarily the food in the water at the season the mussels are harvested. The cycle of plankton bloom is associated with longer days and higher water temperatures, which are affected by vertical currents and not strictly limited to the warmest time of year. And certain detritus and anaerobic material on the bottom can give a less pleasant flavor, so it may matter whether the mussel lived on the bottom or higher up in the water column. But what is most important is what the mussels have eaten lately.

The crunch encountered in eating some mussels is either sand or tiny incipient pearls. The pearl develops when a microscopic parasite (harmless to humans) enters the mussel and the mussel reacts by building a shell around it. Pearls usually take four to five years to grow to noticeable size, so the crunch is rare in farmed mussels. As for sand, bottom-cultured mussels are gathered up in clumps, which are held together by their beards, along with sand and mud, but they are carefully washed and then purged in tanks of seawater so that they disgorge their grit.

Generally, it is best to buy farmed mussels because they are fatter and younger. They show their youth by their blacker, smoother shells with sharper edges. The slower-growing wild mussel puts on a thicker, rougher shell, whose black is gradually worn away to show blue or silver. Barnacles typically have time to establish themselves on the shell, and must be scraped off when the mussel is cleaned. At the fish market, wild or farmed mussels, like other seafood, should be sitting directly on ice. Besides buying from a conscientious market with an overriding concern for freshness, you may be able to ask for a specific brand of farmed mussel that has proven good. (It's uncomfortable to ask questions at a fish counter when the answers reveal that the store has deficiencies, but presumably there would be more good fish markets if consumers weren't too timid to speak up.)

In taste, there is no great advantage to small over large mussels or the reverse, though the small ones may be tenderer. (For what it is worth, the French market, most demanding in the world, prefers small ones. The French will pay more for quality than the Belgians will, but the Belgians are very adept mussel cooks and perhaps more enthusiastic ones.) It isn't clear why some mussel flesh is more orange and other beige; color seems unrelated to taste. But avoid spawning mussels because they are meager, the cooked meats nearly miniature in the shell. The timing of the natural harvest season depends on the part of the world. Fortunately, mussel farmers normally stagger the seeding and don't harvest from spawning beds, so spawning mussels don't find their way into good stores.

Nearly every seafood cookbook contains the obsolete advice that mussels should be bought with beards still attached because debearding harms them. Actually, only when a beard is forcibly pulled is the mussel hurt; thus, beards should be cut. When farmed mussels are cleaned and purged in great tanks, they are intentionally shaken up to encourage them to release their beards, which most do. It is as if, in nature, they were preparing to reattach themselves to the shore after a storm. If you buy mussels with beards, you almost certainly have wild mussels.

Mussels should be eaten as soon as possible after they are harvested. They may last for several days if they are kept cool, but their flavor steadily declines. Fresh mussels, like other fresh seafood, don't smell fishy, but a live mussel that has been out of the water too long both smells and tastes fishy. An American mussel farmer who also operates in Europe says French supermarkets consider the shelf life of a mussel to be twenty-four hours; the time in US supermarkets is seven days. Between purchase and cooking, mussels should be kept very cold in an open container, never a sealed plastic bag: they must breathe. In the refrigerator, mussels survive best in a colander with ice over them for added cold and humidity, and with a pan beneath to catch water.

A very fresh mussel, wild or cultured, remains tightly shut. A mussel gapes only when the adductor muscle that holds it closed tires and weakens, and the hinge on the shell swings open. Avoid buying mussels that gape. And certainly any gaping mussel that doesn't slowly close when it is knocked or agitated should be thrown out.

Even though the shellfish industry is carefully regulated in the US, in light of ocean pollution some people shy away from eating any raw fish or shellfish. But exceptionally plump, fresh farmed mussels are occasionally eaten raw like oysters. Many of the mussels sold on the East Coast are farmed in the cold, relatively clean waters off Maine and are as safe as any raw seafood. I don't particularly care for raw mussels, and none of the New England mussel farmers I've talked to eat them raw, unless it is to check on quality.

Usually, in preparing any dish the first step is to cook the mussels to open them, but occasionally mussels are shucked raw to avoid cooking them twice. To shuck: hold the mussel over a bowl to catch any juices and carefully slip a knife between the shells to cut the adductor muscle, which is near the rounded end of the shell. Mussels are much easier to open than oysters.

The ideal is to cook the mussel just until it withdraws from lining the shell and forms an ellipse. Overcooking causes the mussel to shrink further, expelling more juices and becoming tough. The classical French style is to remove the dark, bandlike gill surrounding the mussel after cooking on the theory that it is slightly tough, but that's unnecessary with a cultured mussel. For formal presentation, small mussel meats can be arranged two to a shell. To be sure of avoiding sand, pass the cooking juices through a cloth-lined strainer. Allow about one pound of mussels in their shells per person (a dozen to a dozen and a half mussels, depending on their size), more for big eaters and mussel lovers, taking into account that a pound of well-farmed mussels contains more meat than a pound of almost any wild ones.

Mussels, rich in protein, contain little fat. Frequent components of mussel dishes are spinach, tomato, bacon or ham, and saffron. Mixtures served in the shell may be covered with bread crumbs and browned under a broiler. Mussels often appear with other seafood and sometimes with meats, as in modern versions of Spanish paella. Some easy preparations are mussels with pasta and mussels served cool, marinated in a vinaigrette. A recipe of the great chef Fernand Point (1897–1955) calls for mussels, butter, cream, a thickening of egg yolk, and a garnish of croutons, showing that the lean essence of mussel flavor can be set off merely by dairy richness. The combination is calculated, but Fernand Point was devoted to richness: *"Du beurre! Donnez-moi du beurre! Toujours du beurre!"*

For drink, a Muscadet from the Loire is a reflexive but excellent choice. The very best Muscadets offer more of the mild fruit flavor of the Muscadet grape, which, together with the wine's clean, lively, refreshing lightness, makes it a successful accompaniment to crustaceans and shellfish. A Muscadet should come from the most recent vintage available. Another good choice is a pilsner or amber beer, or a spicy, hoppy Belgian beer, which is the popular drink with mussels in Belgium, where there is so much enthusiasm for this shellfish.

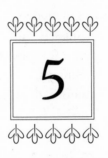

Sorrel, Wild and Tame

In the field, at the edge of the garden by the farmhouse where we used to live, tender wild sorrel grew a dozen feet away from a row of the cultivated kind. Both sorts offer an underused and stimulating tartness. Sorrel is sour like lemon, but without citrus overtones; the tartness is vegetable, as you would expect from a potherb. A private garden and nature used to be almost the only places to find sorrel in the United States, but now sorrel is grown in market gardens and greenhouses and is increasingly available in supermarkets year-round.

Sorrel appears most often in soup and sauce, but it has wide application. Raw, the leaves are strikingly pleasant in a mixture of salad greens. There is such a thing as a purée of buttered sorrel, but often a small amount of sorrel is mixed with a more central ingredient. It enters a stuffing for fish or veal, a gratin with spinach, a mousse, soufflé, omelette, even a custard. Eggs in many forms go well with sorrel. A fish may appear on a bed of sorrel. A sizable quantity is needed to foil the salt richness of sausage.

Sorrel enlivens soup, such as a simple combination of lentils, sorrel, and cream. I especially like a soup of lentils, red wine, duck stock, spinach, and sorrel. The most famous and classical sorrel soup, *potage Germiny*, is enriched with cream and egg yolks.

Wild and tame sorrels as well as spinach take much of their

flavor from oxalic acid. But sorrel is more sour and spinach is more astringent, and they combine well. When sorrel leaves are torn up for salad, they should join a combination of more neutral components as well as other assertive ones — rocket, hyssop, mustard leaves, nasturtium flowers and leaves, and, if possible, chervil leaves. Both chervil and chives are useful garnishes for sorrel dishes.

Apart from soup, in most preparations sorrel starts out as purée. The leaves are washed of grit (a large bowl of water, changed as needed, is more effective than a running tap), and the stems are pulled off backwards, like spinach stems, to carry away any coarse veins. Then about two dozen leaves at a time are laid parallel in a neat pile, rolled into a fat cigar, and the compressed leaves are shredded crosswise with a knife. The shreds go into a pan with a generous teaspoon of butter — or a little water, olive oil, or cream — to a quarter pound of leaves. Over low heat with occasional stirring, they melt into a purée in about fifteen minutes. Don't be dismayed that the heat instantly turns the sorrel from bright green to olive drab. That is the inevitable effect of the acid. Sorrel is cooked in a noncorrosive pot because otherwise the strong acid draws out potentially harmful compounds with very unpleasant metallic tastes. If the ensuing dish is to be elegant or if the leaves are coarse, the purée is put through a fine strainer. Sometimes the sauce needs to be drained or reduced. An addition of cream makes the purée into sauce. The usual seasonings are only salt and pepper.

With sorrel, the cook must be sensitive to balance. Salt or fat calms its temper (from a few spoonfuls to much more cream or crème fraîche, butter, goose fat). In lieu of those, the acid can be offset with a distinctive flavor from another source or with the unctuousness of rich meat juices or stock. Or sorrel can be diluted with the starch of dried beans or potato. (Curiously, Escoffier's interest in starches, especially in the shortcomings of flour as a binder for classic sauces, led him to pay uncommon attention to the range of starches that can give balance and consistency to sorrel soups. His *Guide culinaire* lists smooth sorrel *crèmes* and purées thickened by semolina, vermicelli, sago, tapioca, buckwheat, oatmeal, and barley. He attributes to each variation its own traits. But during the 1970s and 1980s, such starch-thickened soups and sauces fell into disgrace, accused of an unsophisticated and unhealthful heaviness. Yet in the hands of a skilled cook, starch-bound soups and sauces were never thick and gloppy. They were always good.)

Rather than diluting sorrel with starch or playing off another flavor against its sharp edge, you can subdue it by combining it with lettuce. For soup, I like a loosely packed cup of shredded sorrel to three cups of shredded lettuce. Cook three or four scallions in butter over low heat until they are soft but not brown. Add the sorrel and let it melt to a purée, then add the lettuce, which will retain more of its texture. Pass the cooked vegetables through a food mill or whirl them briefly in a food processor or blender. Return them to the stove with two cups of poultry stock and bring this nearly to a boil. Last, pour in a cup of light or heavy cream and season with salt and pepper. Heat the soup without boiling or the cream will separate in the presence of the acid.

The leaves of garden sorrel (*Rumex acetosa*) are arrowhead shaped, the large points at the base running parallel to the stem. Leaves that are only a few weeks old are much tenderer and less sour than older ones. To remove some acid, leaves can be parboiled and drained before use. Older leaves reach ten inches. Leaves up to about six inches long are young enough and of a practical size when a pound or two are needed.

In the garden, pick the leaves one at a time, and if you fall behind as the summer passes (as you almost certainly will), cut the plants off at the ground; they will quickly push up new leaves. The whole plant rises over three feet tall, counting the flowering stalks, which should be cut out as they insistently reappear; the many small, unimpressive reddish flowers are no loss. (I recently saw in the uncultivated soil of a poorly tended garden that sorrel generously self-sows after it flowers; a mass of green seedlings outlined each fallen stalk.) My garden soil is enriched, but sorrel does adequately without that. It stands neglect, although, without cutting, the steady supply of foliage will stop. In northern gardens, sorrel likes full sun, but in the South, part shade may help. Sorrel is a very hardy perennial, one of the first plants to show in spring, when for a few weeks it has little taste. I have grown it easily both from seed and from divisions given to me by another gardener. Twice, in a few years' time I have extended a small clump into a ten-foot row.

More than half a dozen kinds of wild sorrel grow in different parts of North America, and they are easy to identify with the help of a wildflower book. Most grow on open land, often in the otherwise inhospitable areas called waste places; their presence generally indicates poor and acid soil. The wild sorrel that grew in the sandy soil outside my garden was sheep sorrel (R. acetosella). Its leaves are no more than two inches long; they have the same arrowhead shape as garden sorrel, except the lobes at the base splay outward from the stem. Like other naturalized Old World herbs, sheep sorrel is often said to have come to America as a weed mixed in with other seed or with hay brought over from Europe to feed shipboard animals. But those who have studied the colonial use of herbs say such herbs were intentionally planted. The native wild sorrels were gathered by Indians before the arrival of the first European settlers, who in turn used them, along with the species newly introduced from Europe.

The wood sorrels — common, violet, yellow, and others — belong to the genus Oxalis (Latin for both "garden sorrel" and "sour wine"). The mostly low-growing, delicate plants can be told by their cloverlike leaves. The flowers, some quite pretty, vary from less than half an inch up to an inch across. Yellow wood sorrel, O. europea, is the most common wood sorrel where I live, and despite its botanical name it is an American native. It grows in open woods, fields, and even lawns. Since wood sorrel leaves are only half to three-quarters of an inch wide, they are difficult to gather in quantity and best used as garnishes or in salad. Wood sorrel was once obligatory in Julienne, the soup of mixed vegetables and broth or water. The soup gave its name both to the vegetables in it and to their particular shape of short, square-cut sticks about a quarter of an inch wide. The vegetables are supposed to have been modeled on the stems of wood sorrel, which unlike the leaves did not dissolve, remaining visible in the soup. The soup was made as long ago as the eighteenth century, and no one knows who Julien or Julienne was.

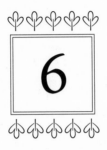

6

The Atlantic Salmon

These days there is plenty of fresh salmon to eat in North America — wild from the Pacific or farmed from either coast, and from Scotland, Chile, the Norwegian fjords, and elsewhere — all readily flown to destinations too far away for rapid trucking. There is only one Atlantic salmon, the classically admired *Salmo salar*, native to both Europe and America. Whereas five kinds of salmon live on the North American side of the Pacific. And the thirty-four thousand miles of Alaska coast harbor 90 percent of US wild salmon, with Alaskan salmon constituting a third of the world's wild salmon harvest. The 1990 catch of Alaska salmon was 140 million fish, a resurgence through careful management from fewer than 100 million ten years before. But in the United States, among all the salmon it is very rare ever to find for sale a fresh wild Atlantic salmon.

It is the fate of all salmon to be anadromous — fish that run (from the Greek *anádromos*, "running upward"). They are born in fresh water, but as adults they live in the sea and then return one or more years later to spawn in the freshwater streams of their birth. Sturgeon, shad, alewives, blueback herring, and smelt are all anadromous. (In a curious inversion, the catadromous American eel lives mostly in fresh water and spawns in salt water; males and females find their way to the Sargasso Sea, where they mate, and where they meet the very similar European eel, which mates there as well.) Somewhat incredibly, a salmon finds its way back to the precise stream of its birth by smell. When the young swim to the sea for the first time, they record the particular chemical scent, derived from plants and minerals, of their natal streams and other waters they pass through on the way to the ocean; the process is called sequential imprinting. What explains the salmon's ability to find their way in the open ocean is less certain. According to the leading theory, salmon navigate by the sun, moon, stars, and the weak magnetic force of the earth. However they manage at sea, when salmon are ready to spawn they select their particular river and make their way home by repeating the sequential imprint in reverse. Only a tiny number of salmon ever err and travel up the wrong river.

In its power and proportions, its speed, agility, patience, and endurance, the salmon is a fish designed for the upriver struggle. It is dark above and light below with shining silver sides that seem to show it off, though its coloring is ocean camouflage. *Salmo salar* is "salmon the leaper." The Atlantic salmon will hurl itself to the top of a dam or falls ten feet tall or a little higher, if there is a deep pool from which to take its start. The average Atlantic salmon is twenty to forty inches long and weighs from four to twenty pounds, although once the fish commonly grew much larger. With its power and abilities and its culinary charms, it satisfies strong human appetites for both food and sport. In Izaak Walton's phrase, it is "the King of freshwater fish."

Many salmon, called grilse, are ready to return and spawn after only one year at sea, but some salmon wait at least two years, and a smaller number wait longer. Then instinct drives the mature, well-fattened salmon homeward. As Walton wrote, "though they make very hard shift to get out of the fresh rivers into the sea, yet they will make harder shift to get out of the salt into the fresh rivers, to spawn, or possess the pleasures that they have formerly found in them: to which end, they will force themselves through floodgates, or over weirs, or hedges, or stops in the water, even to a height beyond common belief." He quotes the somewhat fantastic vision of the poet Michael Drayton. The salmon

> *His tail takes in his mouth, and, bending like a bow*
> *That's to full compass drawn, aloft himself doth throw,*
> *Then springing at his height, as doth a little wand*
> *That bended end to end, and started from man's hand,*
> *Far off itself doth cast; so does that Salmon vault.*

The salmon indeed arches itself to thrust against the water, and Walton's understanding of breeding is close enough to the modern one. "He is said to breed or cast his spawn, in most rivers, in the month of August: some say, that then they dig a hole or grave in a safe place in the gravel, and there place their eggs or spawn, after the melter has done his natural office, and then hide it most cunningly, and cover it over with gravel and stones; and leave it to their Creator's protection, who, by a gentle heat which he infuses into that cold element, makes it brood, and beget life in the spawn, and to become Samlets early in the spring next following."

When the salmon reaches fresh water, it ceases to feed and begins to live on its stored fat. But, for a reason that no one can explain, the fasting salmon will seize an angler's fly. Some salmon, Atlantic or Pacific, spawn not far from the mouth of a river, but others swim hundreds of miles inland. Certain salmon in the Pechora River in northern Russia travel a thousand miles, overwintering and nearly reaching the Ural Mountains. During the river journey, a salmon's strength is drawn into developing milt or roe; the fish takes on a darkish coloring (red in Pacific salmon), and the male's lower jaw juts forward in an ugly hook. With the onset of these changes, salmon make poor eating. On the upstream climb, they periodically rest behind rocks or wait for a greater or lesser flow of water to help them past obstacles. When they reach an acceptable gravelly shallow, the female digs a nest four to twelve inches deep with her tail. Into it a ten-pound fish, for example, releases seven to eight thousand orange eggs the size of a large pea. These are fertilized by one or several males and buried under gravel. The spent salmon are called kelts, and after the ordeal most Atlantic salmon die (as all Pacific salmon do). Some survive to return to the ocean, and a few kelts spawn again another year; a tiny number thereafter.

Early the next spring, the eggs hatch into half-inch-long alevins with their yolk sacs still attached; about four weeks later, when the food in the yolk is gone, these become fry, which emerge from the gravel and swim about the nest; at about two and a half inches, distinctive dark "parr marks" appear on their sides along with small red spots, and for the next two or three years, sometimes as many as six, they will be parr — until at last one spring they undergo a rapid transformation. They become smolts with silvery adult coloring. Still only three to six inches long, the smolts promptly swim down to the sea on the spring flood. At each stage, the young salmon find enemies. The eggs are a delicacy for trout. Cormorants, herons, gulls, kingfishers, eels, trout, perch, and other fish feast on the salmon later on. The upshot of eight thousand original eggs may be as few as two adults.

Before Europeans settled in North America, the continent's number of Atlantic salmon was anywhere from less than two million to nearly ninety million, by various modern estimates. Of course, hardly any of these fish were caught. The native American peoples valued and some venerated the salmon, but the predations of their tiny populations scarcely mattered in light of the tremendous supply. According to the Norse sagas, when the Vikings reached Vinland a thousand years ago, "There was no lack of salmon either in the river or in the lake, and larger salmon than they had ever seen before." That is strong testimony from people who knew their salmon well.

The stories of superabundant fish of all kinds in the early days would hardly be credible except that they bear each other out. When, a few years after Columbus's first voyages, Sebastian Cabot said there were so many fish in the Saint Lawrence that they slowed his father's boat, the exaggeration may have been slight. As late as the 1800s, there were rivers where men drove wagons into the water and filled them with salmon using pitchforks. More than a dozen rivers and streams in North America are named Salmon or Salmon Falls. During the runs, salmon were preserved in brine, salted in barrels, sometimes smoked.

Yet in 1990, exactly 263 Atlantic salmon were counted in the Connecticut River in their annual run upstream to spawn — a cruelly small number compared with the multitudes that once clogged the rivers of North America and Europe. Salmon have been barred from river after river by dams, or their waters have been poisoned by pollution. Otherwise, if it were possible to eliminate salmon from a river solely by catching every one (and it may be), they would have disappeared in many places through extreme overfishing, with weirs or nets sometimes stretched across whole watercourses.

Truly, that any salmon at all could be counted in the Connecticut is an encouraging event after the devastation of the last three hundred years. Likely, the two greatest salmon rivers of the eastern United States were once the Connecticut and Maine's Penobscot, guessing from historical reports and from the lengths of the rivers and their tributaries. In the 1700s, the Connecticut was the more famous for its salmon. It is slightly longer, 402 miles measured from Long Island Sound north through Connecticut, Massachusetts, Vermont, and New Hampshire to its headwaters in New Hampshire's Connecticut Lakes, near the Quebec border. In times past, salmon are believed to have reached the first of these lakes. In *The Atlantic Salmon: A Vanishing Species*, Anthony Netboy recounts the history of the despoliation of the salmon, country by country. In the eighteenth century at the mouth of the Connecticut, "It was possible to catch 3,700 salmon in one haul in Old Saybrook's South Cove." Yet, "when a solitary salmon strayed into the Connecticut in 1872 the Saybrook fishermen, never having seen this fish, could not identify it!"

In fact, the river had hardly seen salmon for fifty years. The first dam to completely block the main stem of the Connecticut River was built at Turners Falls, Massachusetts, in 1798; it was sixteen feet tall, several feet higher than any salmon can jump. The early small dams for gristmills and sawmills posed little problem for salmon. But as the Industrial Revolution gained force, ever taller dams were built lower and lower down main sections of wide rivers. In 1837 in Maine, the Kennebec, which had great runs of salmon, was dammed at Augusta, reducing the accessible length of the river from three hundred miles to fifty. In 1847 a dam built across the Merrimack River at Lawrence, Massachusetts, cut off all spawning grounds. When an impassable dam was built, the fish would still return every year and gather below, each time in smaller numbers, until after about a decade they ceased to come again. Large river systems were commonly filled with several dozen dams of all sizes, almost none of them passable. Besides barring fish, a dam may flood salmon habitat upstream or change the nature of the watercourse downstream by trapping silt or reducing the flow.

On the Pacific coast, the Columbia River once provided more spawning grounds for salmon than any other river in the world. There were runs in every month of the year. The 550-foot-tall Grand Coulee Dam, begun in 1933, alone cut off perhaps half the river's habitat. With later dams and other degradation, the runs today are pathetically reduced.

The salmon enthusiast's solution to the problem of a dam, though not one as tall as the Grand Coulee, is some kind of fish passage up and down, offering help to all kinds of anadromous fish. As long ago as 1318 the Scottish parliament required an opening in dams to allow smolts to pass downstream, and many subsequent laws and regulations elsewhere, especially from the nineteenth century onward, have required fish passages. But until fairly recently the laws were mostly ignored or defied. Many of the fish ladders that were built were so poorly designed that they did not work at all; some of those are still being replaced. Possibly half of all New England dams do not yet have them. Very tall dams require lifts — fish elevators. Today, the best fish ladder is 90 percent effective, which sounds reassuring until you multiply it dam by dam. A salmon that encounters the five large dams now open on the Connecticut (several major dams remain closed upstream) has only a 60 percent chance of getting through them all (a dozen ladders, not unheard of, would reduce this to 25 percent, and those figures assume the fish find the ladders). It was once believed that fish didn't need help in traveling downstream. But the mortality rate of fish going through the turbines of a hydroelectric plant may average 10 to 15 percent, depending on the turbines. The fish can be protected from that if they are diverted to a spillway or otherwise guided to safety, but in many places this remains to be done. As the head of the Maine Atlantic Salmon Commission told me, "We are in dire need of state-of-the-art upstream and downstream fish passage facilities."

In North America, the Atlantic salmon's natural range extends as far north as the rivers flowing into the Ungava Bay in Quebec, west of the coast of Labrador, and southward it takes in all of Atlantic Canada and New England through the state of Connecticut, where historically salmon regularly entered the Housatonic, only fifty miles from Manhattan. Besides anadromous salmon, landlocked Atlantic salmon — isolated by the disruptions and retreat of the glaciers — occur in a few lakes in New England, Canada, Scandinavia, and Russia. There was once a vast number of nonseagoing salmon in Lake Ontario, and today the population is rebounding.

On the European side of the Atlantic, salmon formerly thrived in rivers from Portugal — where salmon are no longer found at all — all the way north and east past Norway to the Russian rivers flowing into the Barents and Kara seas. Salmon ran plentifully in the rivers of the British Isles and of Iceland. The names of European rivers that formerly held salmon form practically a list of the great rivers of Europe: the Seine, the Moselle, the Thames (the last of the original salmon was caught in 1833, but happily salmon have been reintroduced), the Rhine (which died from pollution a century ago; efforts are on to restore it), the Elbe, the Douro in Portugal, the Oder in Poland. Of France, Anthony Netboy says, "No other country in Europe, probably, was better endowed with inland fisheries — and none frittered them away so completely." Some salmon are still seen in the Loire and in the Adour, which descends from the Pyrenees, and in smaller rivers in Brittany and Normandy. Restoration of the Loire and Allier is under way. The Mediterranean is too warm for salmon, and it may be inhospitable for other reasons.

Because the salmon is so well loved for its sport and its taste, and has so much economic value as a food source, efforts to protect it began at an impressively early date. The first fishing regulations were enacted under Charlemagne in the eighth or ninth century. In 1030, Malcolm II of Scotland established a late-summer closed season for salmon, and in the 1200s England began to restrict fishing and punish poachers. By the nineteenth century, efforts at conservation were widespread. If all that was enacted had been carried out, the salmon might have prospered wherever the water remained unpolluted.

Of course, the best surroundings for the small brooks that most salmon favor is the protective cover of primeval forest, not clear land. Maine, home of almost all surviving US Atlantic salmon, suffered especially from logging. Clear-cutting reduces the capacity of the land to hold water, so that storms create sudden washes that flush eggs and fry from streams; in dry times, low water levels drop still further. Erosion from logging roads fills streams with silt, covering the salmon's needed clean gravel. And the giant Maine log drives gouged streambeds. Sawdust and other logging waste were dumped into streams along with untreated waste from pulp mills; the waste takes so much oxygen from water that fish cannot live.

By the 1880s, regular runs of salmon appeared in only seven Maine rivers. The average commercial catch was still 150,000 pounds a year, but it fell rapidly. By 1910 the only rivers in Maine — the only rivers in the United States — with significant runs of Atlantic salmon were the Dennys, the Saint Croix, and the Penobscot. All declined, and by the late 1950s the number of salmon in the Penobscot had dropped almost to zero. The most southerly salmon left in the East were a third of the way up the Maine coast in the Sheepscot.

Happily, today the Penobscot run has been assiduously built

back up to three to five thousand fish, and the hope is to increase this in about a decade to between eight and twelve thousand. Farther east in Maine, five small rivers, where currently neither dams nor water quality is a problem, have minor runs of two hundred to four hundred salmon, making a total of seven salmon rivers plus eight under restoration.

Even when salmon were nearly eliminated from the United States, they were relatively abundant in many of their several hundred Canadian rivers. Some rivers suffered serious declines in the nineteenth century, but the number of Atlantic salmon in Canada in the twentieth century remained greater than in any other country.

The Atlantic salmon has been studied in earnest for a hundred years, and the volume of information has accelerated in recent decades. Much about migration at sea has been learned by tagging the fish, with the cooperation of fishermen who retrieve the tags. The scales of a salmon show seasonal rings of growth that reveal age, number of times of spawning, and length of time spent at sea. Study of DNA confirms that there are three great races of Atlantic salmon — American, European, and Baltic — and within them each river's salmon form a separate genetic strain, at least two thousand strains of *Salmo salar* altogether. Even within a river, the salmon of different tributaries differ from one another. Each group is believed to be specially adapted to surviving in the particular conditions of its home waters. Naturally, only a stock of larger and fatter fish will swim up a river's distant reaches, but far more subtle traits may make it difficult or impossible for a strain to get established in alien waters, as experimenters have sometimes tried to do. This inadaptation is a problem when a river loses its salmon. The strain is then extinct, and to restore salmon to the river, a new strain must be created, which has been done successfully in some rivers. But in large river systems like the Connecticut, where there are multiple dams and other problems, the combination of human assistance and natural selection is slow-acting and costly.

For the Connecticut, salmon eggs were begged from agencies in Maine and Canada, and some were taken from landlocked salmon in binational Lake Memphremagog in Vermont and Quebec. Sperm came mostly from Penobscot salmon in Maine. Most of the returning fish each year are still taken from the Connecticut to provide eggs and sperm for next year's crop of hatchery fish. It is only just conceivable that any salmon are yet reproducing in the river itself.

So far, over half the length of the Connecticut and many more miles of tributaries have been reopened to anadromous fish. Although the size of the runs remains low, with the number of salmon remaining in the hundreds, someday the self-sustaining population could reach tens or hundreds of thousands. No one knows how many salmon the modern river can support, though certainly many fewer than it once did. The quality of water in northeastern rivers improved starting about 1980, and some dams have been removed, but with the pressure for nonpolluting (especially nonpetroleum) sources of electric power, hydroelectric dams continue to receive support. In addition, as farmland and forest in the watershed are taken for development, more water is taken from the river for drinking, waste treatment, and industry. Some, too, goes for agriculture.

Another problem in the short term is that very roughly half (no one knows for certain) of US-born Atlantic salmon are fished in the ocean before they ever have a chance to spawn. US salmon join Canadian salmon in feeding grounds off Newfoundland and Labrador, where commercial fishing continues, although it is slowly being phased out. Some salmon from both countries then swim on to summer feeding grounds in the Davis Strait off the west coast of Greenland. There they are joined by salmon from some parts of Europe. This arctic and subarctic feeding pattern was discovered in the 1950s and unfortunately starting in 1957 gave rise to a commercial fishery off Greenland. Another concentration of European salmon was found north of the Faeroe Islands between Scandinavia and Iceland, and this began to be exploited heavily in the late 1970s. From the Greenland fishery, 227 metric tons of salmon were taken in

1990 — well below the agreed-upon limit but still far too high. The North Atlantic Salmon Conservation Organization in Edinburgh is negotiating to end all ocean interception of salmon. The eventual goal is that fishing of Atlantic salmon will take place entirely in individual rivers so that fish stocks can be monitored and conserved.

With all the recent activity on behalf of the salmon, the situation as a whole is encouraging but still mixed. Some strong runs of Atlantic salmon occur in Scotland, Ireland, Norway, Sweden, and Canada. But much more can be done in these countries, and the natural runs are often supplemented with stocking by hatcheries. The strongest overall runs are in Iceland and northern Russia.

Many fish, although delectable when impeccably fresh and cooked to perfect doneness, have comparatively little flavor. The flavor and texture that are so much appreciated in the salmon are partly due to the fish's fat, including the fat's moistening effect. In a salmon steak the alternating rings of light fat and pink muscle are plainly visible as is the concentrated fat in the belly flap. A too-fat farmed fish tastes unpleasantly oily, and farmed salmon has a lingering reputation for being fatty. Farmed Atlantic salmon has become commonplace, but before considering it more closely, it is worth knowing something of the Pacific salmon, the wild salmon an American is likeliest to eat.

With five species covering an immense range from California to Alaska, the diversity of wild Pacific salmon stands in pointed contrast to Atlantic salmon. The two most highly regarded Pacific salmon are king, or chinook, and sockeye — both of them far more esteemed by many West Coast enthusiasts than Atlantic salmon are. They are rich in fat, averaging roughly 10 percent. The king, most often favored (an Alaska king can provide forty pounds of steaks), has brilliant orange-red flesh, although there are some white-fleshed Alaska kings. It is disputed whether pigment has any connection to flavor, which clearly varies within the species according to time of year and the place where the fish are taken. The disagreement over which salmon is best stems partly from geographic rivalry. Besides species, the important real difference among salmon is the length of river journey a salmon is prepared for — as shown by its fat.

West Coast salmon are not *Salmo* at all but *Oncorhynchus*, "hooknose." As a proud Alaskan says, "We still don't consider the Atlantic salmon a salmon anyway." But there are many partisans of the Atlantic salmon, the classical fish. (Pliny said, "The river salmon surpasses all the fishes of the sea.") Hal Lyman, former publisher of *Saltwater Sportsman* magazine, shortly after he returned from salmon fishing on the Kola Peninsula in Russia, told me, "I don't think Pacific salmon can touch Atlantic salmon." It seems that the taste for Atlantic versus Pacific salmon depends on where you happened to grow up.

Unlike wild salmon, farmed Atlantic salmon is available all year, and the size and the quality from a single producer scarcely vary. That helps to guarantee a large share of the market. And farmed salmon is not at all to be disparaged. Of all farmed fish, a well-raised Atlantic salmon is probably the closest to wild. Even some people who have done a lot of fishing say the two types taste the same. But farmed salmon isn't a single commodity; it varies according to who raises it and where. It is produced in Norway, Scotland, British Columbia, New Brunswick, Nova Scotia, Washington, Maine, Chile, Tasmania, and more places around the world. The technology of farming, feeding in particular (different feeds produce different results), has greatly improved since salmon were first farmed in Norway in the 1960s. Norway led in developing salmon aquaculture, and methods elsewhere reflect Norwegian ones, though now advances are made everywhere. Among some chefs, Norwegian salmon still has the best reputation.

The freshest salmon you are likely to find on the East Coast is farmed Atlantic salmon, and without freshness, the other points of a fish don't matter. Almost all salmon farmed in the East is raised in the protected coves and inlets along the New Brunswick shore of the Bay of Fundy (the Nova Scotia side is too exposed). A little is raised just outside it in far eastern Maine. Water temperatures in the Bay of Fundy remain unusually steady because the extraordinary high tides — highest in the world — mix warm and cold layers of water. Low tide reveals a vast expanse of reddish shore. Tides that may be six feet at Cape Cod are twenty-five feet or more at the salmon farms in the lower Bay of Fundy. The vertical rise and fall of northeastern tides is greater as the continental shelf grows wider, and the shallowness in the bay continues the effect. Within a bay, tides initiate a kind of bathtub sloshing effect from end to end. If, as in the Bay of Fundy, the timing of the sloshing coincides with the lunar cycle of the tides, then the tides are exaggerated further. At the narrow, shallow head of the bay the water is forced higher still; in its uppermost reaches the tides rise up fifty feet.

On the East Coast, any salmon aquaculture outside the Bay of Fundy is highly chancy because the water is either too warm or too cold or both. Salmon are killed at a temperature just below freezing. In winter, the bay is warmer than the adjacent open ocean, and in summer it is cooler than more southern waters, which grow too warm for salmon. Also, the Fundy tides stir up nutrients from the cold bottom into warmer water, where they sustain a rich mix of aquatic life. The lower part of the bay is the only spot close in to the shore in North America where shoals of wild salmon spend the winter.

In October 1990, I visited the Bay of Fundy to see a few of the fifty-seven salmon farms and to speak with Dr. John Anderson of the Atlantic Salmon Federation, one of the two leading private organizations devoted to conserving the wild Atlantic salmon. The ASF also assists aquaculture through genetic research so as to take commercial pressure off the wild fish. The group is located in Chamcook, New Brunswick, a short drive from the Maine border.

Its buildings are next to, and partly in, the small Chamcook Creek, recently restored to salmon by creating passage around an old milldam. Actually in the creek is a visitors' center with exhibits, including live salmon at different ages. Nearby, dozens of round tanks covered with green netting hold experiments in salmon breeding; more tanks are indoors. The experimental salmon, like all the region's aquaculture salmon, come originally from the Saint John River strain, already well adapted to the bay. The ASF provides genetically selected brood stock to commercial hatcheries that raise smolts for the farms. To compete in the market, the farms want salmon that grow to eight to ten pounds in eighteen months without reaching sexual maturity. And those salmon should be resistant to disease.

The advent of farming brings a new kind of interference with nature. John Anderson of the ASF is concerned in part about diseases introduced back and forth between wild and domestic salmon. "I just learned a couple of weeks ago that nine rivers in Norway are epidemically infected with furunculosis. Some of these are famous salmon rivers; one seems to be about to lose its salmon altogether." The cause is infected fish imported from Scotland. Another concern is the effect of escaped farm salmon, no longer adapted to the wild. They are thought to interbreed readily with wild fish; if so, they would dilute the natural gene pool. The wild population is now 30 to 40 percent escapees in some Norwegian rivers. "Some people say not to worry. We just don't know." But if the problem of dilution is serious, it will be a long time before it is corrected. And some conservationists find a philosophical or aesthetic drawback to no longer having pure strains of wild salmon. Another adversity is the effect of acid rain, which can lower the pH of fresh water beyond the tolerance of salmon. "For the wild stocks acid rain is quite a serious problem. There are thirteen rivers in Nova Scotia that have lost their salmon and eighteen others that are threatened." The problem is worse in Sweden and Norway.

However, most of my conversation with John Anderson was not about difficulties, and he is more than optimistic. Problems are what make research exciting. On farmed salmon: "To me it tastes great. The main reason may be the fish really are fresh."

About twenty miles east of Chamcook is the town of Saint

George, where on the day of my arrival the high tide was twenty-six feet seven inches. Just before the road enters town, it crosses the Magaguadavic River, where a long concrete fish ladder climbs a rock wall to pass over a dam. Beyond the town toward the water is the processing plant owned by Sea Farm Canada, which raises and sells smolts to a number of farmers and is the second-largest producer of salmon at several sites in the bay.

In the warehouselike processing room, I was surprised to find an absence of fishy smell — only the clean, mineral, oceanic smell of just-killed fish, mixed with the odor of iodine from a pan of disinfectant on the floor (you dip the soles of your shoes in it on entering). The farmed salmon are not fed for two weeks before harvest, which empties their stomachs and firms the flesh. They are killed at the salmon cages on the water three to four hours before they arrive in Saint George. They are transported in an icy slush in gray plastic tubs about four feet square. Prompt chilling keeps fish fresher longer and reduces the effects of rigor mortis. The processing that goes on here is simply gutting and then packing whole salmon with ice in smaller boxes for shipping to wholesalers; for a few orders, a specialized machine slices salmon into steaks. Nearly all salmon raised in the Bay of Fundy is sold fresh rather than frozen. Harvest and shipping are highly organized, and, in theory, thirty-six hours later the salmon can be served at dinner in San Francisco.

From Sea Farm, we drove down to the water. At the end of a gravel road by Finger Cove is the smaller plant of Jail Island Salmon, which raises and sells about a hundred thousand salmon a year. The company is owned by George Wolf, known as Skip, and his large, ebullient partner, Wally Balasiuk, former Toronto Argonaut. The farm was begun in 1981 by Skip and his wife, Karen, with other partners who fell away before Wally joined them; only two farms on the bay started earlier (the first, an experimental one in 1978). When I opened the door, Skip and eight young men with thin knives were cleaning salmon around a table. Hoses for rinsing hung from the ceiling. Again, no fishy smell. The standard gray tubs held just-killed

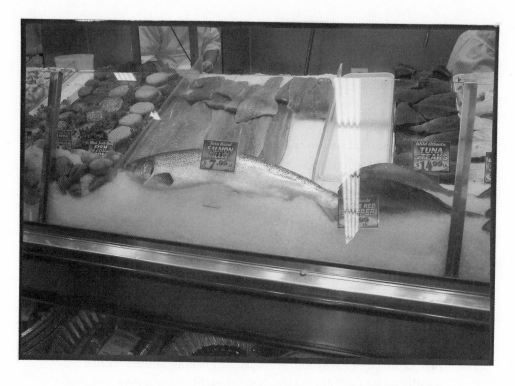

Farm-raised Atlantic salmon at Fairway Market.
New York City, 2004.

salmon in slush. In a few minutes Wally arrived driving a flatbed truck with more full tubs.

I saw most of the plant when I first opened the door. But Wally took me to the smoking room with its stainless-steel smoker from Britain. The smoke comes from hardwood sawdust. The salmon is lightly salted, and Wally says, "I like using the fatter fish." Jail Island smoked salmon is sold only in Canada. We retreated with a smoked filet to the office, where Wally served slices unto repletion and we talked about raising salmon and the ways to eat it. He pointed with his knife to the filet: "My favorite way is right there."

We drove a few minutes along the unspoiled shore to another cove, where three groups of salmon cages were anchored in seventy- to eighty-foot water just offshore (the bottom drops rapidly). Moored nearby were a net-changing machine and a net-cleaning machine for removing seaweed. A boat took us to the cages where five or six workers were harvesting salmon. They are called cages, but they are made of synthetic netting forty feet square at the water's surface and about thirty-six feet deep in the center. When the fish are market size, each contains about forty-five hundred salmon, which regularly jump several feet out of the water. Surrounded by steel-grid walk-ways, each enclosure has stretched over it, perhaps five feet above the water, a wide-meshed net to keep out predators — fish hawks and cormorants — and to keep in serious leapers. A rifle was lying at hand for seals. Once they break into the cages, eating and freeing salmon, seals get a taste for predation and they have to be shot. Wally was apologetic that there isn't a kinder control for what is an expensive problem in the bay.

The fish are caught in a seine and put into one of the gray tubs, where they are stunned by iced water and sometimes by CO_2. They are killed by quickly slitting the gills; then they bleed in another tub continuously flushed with water. Bleeding improves the flavor of fish generally and keeps them fresher longer. The process was neat and not at all macabre. Even in winter the work goes on in the open here at the cages. "You worry about the weather," says Wally. Storms are dangerous for workers and, like seals, they can break cages. But only a rare storm prevents growers from harvesting salmon several times a week every week of the year.

The question of wild versus farmed salmon revolves around feed. Both kinds of fish swim in the same waters. The tides in the Bay of Fundy constantly change the water in the cages and cleanse the bottom, and the fish are continually moving, so they get plenty of exercise if not exactly the same kind as wild fish. Wild Atlantic salmon are opportunistic feeders, predators whose diet reflects the season and the waters where they are. They eat herring, capelin, alewives, needlefish, sand eels, squid, zooplankton, and the shrimp and krill and euphausiids that color their meat orange. Much of this diet is oily fish.

Farmed salmon grow best on a similar diet. The feed, or at least the better feed, is modeled on the wild, and it is supposed to be the most cost-efficient. High-quality feeds are made of fish meal, mostly from the same fish eaten in the wild, mixed with fish oil, mostly from herring and sardines, and with vitamins and minerals and some of the same pigment the wild fish find in crustaceans. All these ingredients are bound with wheat or corn to hold the fish meal together in pellets for the convenience of farmers. Salmon have a good sense of smell and taste, and they will spit out what they don't like, including feed containing catfish, an herbivore. With all the aquaculture in the world, fish feed is big business. One feed manufacturer is Moore-Clark Company (Canada), Inc., in Saint Andrews, New Brunswick. Sam Bowman of the company says, "The salmon tastes like what it eats, and we realize that — and that the salmon grow best in the wild on fish." A moist feed used to be common. It produced more fat and probably gave farmed fish its reputation for oiliness.

Andrew Storey of Sea Farm says, "Farmed fish are fatter than wild fish; there's no question. They grow faster if they're fatter." Of course, what the farmer wants is to produce the most fish from the least feed. The amount of feed is carefully calculated, but reliable figures on the fat content of Atlantic salmon are elusive. With so many variables at work, one expert questions whether it is possible even to generalize about any kind of salmon. Another source, however, says the fat content of farmed salmon varies seasonally from 10 to 15 percent, as opposed to 8 to 10 percent for wild Atlantic salmon. This compares with somewhere around 10 percent for Pacific sockeyes and kings. The issue of whether a wild or a farmed fish is superior may be a false one. In North America, a premium is paid for the top aquaculture salmon. And with all the interplay between wild and domestic, there is some ambiguity about the meaning of wildness. Even the Alaskans increase their salmon numbers with an intermediate practice called ranching.

Smell is a doubtful test at an odoriferous fish counter, but in the sweet air at home, freshness or lack of it is clear enough. I began consistently to select fresher fish from the mixed display at a fish counter when I applied what should have been obvious all along. Beyond having clear eyes, truly fresh whole fish look like live fish; filets look nearly like living flesh. Fresh fish are firm, and the handsome silvery sides of a salmon, especially if it hasn't yet been scaled, have a wet sheen. Fish flesh is delicate; large filets should be supported with two hands so they don't pull apart. Fish should be cooked the day they are bought, and until then they should be kept as near freezing as possible — usually on ice. (The spoilage organisms in fish work at lower temperatures than those in land creatures.) Rinsing a filet before cooking washes away flavor; wipe it instead with a paper towel to catch stray scales, and let heat take care of anything else.

The gastronomic reason we cook food is to alter its taste and its texture. The very best way to appreciate a special salmon is to cook it carefully and simply. (Escoffier: "Salmon is served as plainly as possible … but whatever the method of preparation it is always accompanied by cucumber salad." His recipes show that plainness is a relative concept.) More than with most fish, the pleasure of salmon is its moist yielding texture. The way to ensure that and to retain all the flavorful juices is slow, gentle cooking — such as poaching, starting in cool liquid — so that the outside cooks almost at the same time as the center. Vinegar is often added to a poaching court bouillon for fish, but most vinegar is harsh, muddy, or off-flavored and detracts from the taste of the fish; even tolerable bought vinegar is a rarity. Instead of troubling to make a court bouillon, I like to bake salmon slowly, protected by a parchment cover, in a little mixed wine and water in a 350 degree Fahrenheit oven. With all the variables that affect cooking times, the only way to be certain of doneness is to use a narrow blade to see whether the center of the thickest part has turned opaque or still shows a raw translucence. Bear in mind that a fish in a hot dish will continue to cook gently for several minutes or more after it leaves the oven. To my taste, salmon should be barely cooked in the middle for the best flavor (what in a white-fleshed fish would be faintly pink at the bone). Slowly cooked, salmon is then meltingly tender and separates from the bone with the touch of a fork.

The usual accompaniments to salmon are the ones served with other fish: new potatoes, sorrel (especially with fattier fish), mushrooms, cucumbers, and flavorings of dill, fennel, parsley, lemon, anchovy, green peppercorns, saffron, and capers. A French combination — and an old New England Fourth of July meal, at least around Boston — is salmon and sweet, freshly shelled peas. Salmon and such well-flavored seafood as lobster and monkfish are sometimes given a sybaritic sweet seasoning with vanilla bean, sugar itself, or Sauternes — any of these in a tantalizing, barely identifiable amount. (The combination of vanilla and lobster was made famous by Alain Senderens at the former restaurant Archestrate in Paris; he says the idea came to him when he opened a vanilla pod in Sri Lanka and the aroma reminded him of lobster.) On a more modest plane, the sweet herbal flavors work related changes: chervil, tarragon (in *sauce béarnaise*), fennel, and mint, especially with cream. A very different effect is achieved with a red-wine sauce.

Be aware that the tannin in a glass of red wine can point out a lack of freshness in fish. With rich fish and with bland rich sauces, particularly those hinting at sweet, a full-bodied white wine with some matching sweetness works best. A light wine without sweetness tastes thin and tart.

A delicious dinner of wild salmon is one justification for the restoration of the salmon. But it doesn't explain the extraordinary willingness to spend government and private money to preserve and restore salmon rivers. The motivation is perhaps the sense that salmon are part of a cultural heritage and that they belong in the rivers where they once lived, that something is badly amiss that ought to be corrected. And maybe we want reassurance that environmental harm can be undone. The salmon is a strong, persistent creature whose fate provides a clear measure of the health of land and waters and of how vulnerable we are ourselves. The world's prodigious former runs of salmon were an easily harvested, continually replenished, wholly environmentally benign resource that was squandered. When salmon are eventually restored, a significant economic value will have been regained. And even now there is aesthetic pleasure in a fish that is the angler's ideal, and in the complex ecology that brings so far inland a tangible link to the ocean.

7

Black Pepper

It isn't as ubiquitous as water or salt, but black pepper is probably the third most common addition to food. Pepper is aromatic but not so intensely and distinctly perfumed as the earliest resins and spices used in Arabia before the Arabs had much traffic with lands to either east or west. (They prepared oils and ointments from myrrh, frankincense, and balm.) Nor has pepper the focused flavor of clove, cinnamon, or nutmeg from the Far East. It supplied a more temperate heat in the spice mixtures of Indian cuisines before the arrival of chili peppers from the New World. The most pungent black peppercorns, though they produce a memorable sting in quantity, don't have nearly the force of hot chili peppers. Black pepper was traded in the East long before it was known in the West, but almost from the time it first reached the Continent, it was valued inordinately there. In medieval Europe it was so precious that it was classed with gold, silver, and gems. The desire for pepper led the first European explorers to the New World. Black pepper is still first among spices in quantity produced, about a quarter of the world's total (assuming you count mustard as an herb rather than a spice). Pepper has influenced history and civilization to a degree that is difficult to comprehend.

Black pepper is a sun-dried berry, the fruit of *Piper nigrum*, a climbing vine of the hot wet tropics that grows thirty feet or longer.

It exists in latitudes no farther than twenty degrees either side of the equator and prefers to be closer. Native to India, it grows wild in the Western Ghats, the low mountains that parallel the western coast from the southern tip to north of Bombay. Here, pepper was first cultivated, probably about 1000 BC, and from here a thousand years later it was carried by Hindu immigrants to Malaysia and Indonesia, where it was established in such places as Malacca, Sarawak, Bangka, Java, Sumatra, and the Moluccas (the Spice Islands). In the twentieth century, the plant was introduced as far away as Brazil. But most of the finest black pepper is still that exported from the Malabar Coast of southwestern India.

Black pepper does have relations that are spices, but black, white, and green peppercorns are all fruit of the same plant, colored and flavored differently because they are harvested at different stages of maturity or, in the case of white pepper, stripped of their outer coat. The botanical pepper family does not include the hot chili pepper that Columbus found cultivated on the island of Hispaniola, "which is their pepper, and it is stronger than pepper, and the people won't eat without it." For clarity's sake, chili peppers and the sweet bell peppers are often called capsicums after their genus in the nightshade family. But for a long time Europeans named almost any new aromatic discovery some kind of pepper. Allspice, which was found in the Caribbean, is even now known as pepper in most languages, and it used to be Jamaica pepper in English. Few of these miscellaneous peppers, including Szechuan pepper of the rue family, have any botanical connection to black pepper.

Pepper and other spices, traded through intermediaries, were the earliest connection between East and West, when each scarcely knew of the other. Pepper was known and perhaps used in Greece even before it was brought back by Alexander the Great from his campaign in northern India in the fourth century BC. The important city he founded, Alexandria, was for centuries the major Mediterranean trading center for spices from the East. Spices were carried by boat across the Arabian Sea and up the Red Sea, or they came by way of camel routes to the north. (Similarities in the names of certain spices can be traced from classical Greek to Chinese or Malay, since the names were passed along by traders.) During the first century AD, the Romans learned what the Arabs had long known, to sail across the Arabian Sea with the monsoons to the Malabar Coast; and the Romans began to buy pepper at the Indian source. Still, they were confused about the origin of many other spices, knowing vaguely only of "raftmen," who journeyed from farther east. It may have been at this time, when black pepper was plentiful and ceased to be a luxury, that it was first regarded as an essential spice anywhere in the West. It is the most common seasoning in the recipes of the Roman epicure Apicius, added in the kitchen and again at the table. Black pepper became the leading Roman spice, used far into the empire's European provinces.

But as Rome declined and the Islamic Empire spread across the Mediterranean into Spain, Europeans lost what knowledge they had had of the origins of spices. It is often said that Arab traders kept the sources secret, but in any case Europeans were in no position to trade across the seas. After Alexandria, a last remnant of the old Roman Empire, fell in 641 AD, few spices appear to have penetrated far into Europe until after the First Crusade, almost five hundred years later.

Then the thousands of returning pilgrims brought spices back with them. The eastern Mediterranean was again a focus of trade with Europe. And then, although a few Westerners had already traveled to the Far East, the appearance of Marco Polo's exuberant book, written in 1298–99, fired the imagination of Europeans about the lands beyond. Marco Polo reported seeing pepper growing on the Malabar Coast "in great abundance, being found both in the woody and open parts of the country. It is gathered in the months of May, June, and July; and the vines which produce it are cultivated in plantations."

Even now, in Asia pepper is grown largely by small farmers in family plots, hardly more than gardens. In some places in India, the oldest method survives, where a vine is planted at the base of an existing tree and left largely to fend for itself. But here and in other countries the supports are more likely to be trees planted especially for their economic value or for their ability to withstand severe pruning for the sake of the pepper. Under more intensive cultivation, as in Sarawak in Malaysia, rooted cuttings are planted in mounds and shaded temporarily by fern leaves. The ground is kept scrupulously free of weeds, and the vines are attached to stout twelve-foot posts and pruned into fat columns to create a maximum of flowers. The first harvest is taken after three years, and the vines are productive for at least a dozen years more.

The pepper berries are borne on two- to six-inch spikes, fifty to sixty berries on a spike. A berry consists of a fleshy outer layer covering a single seed, which makes the fruit a drupe, like a peach, a cherry, or an olive. The harvest lasts several months, since the spikes don't all ripen at once. Ripe pepper berries are red. For black pepper, the spikes are picked when the berries are full-sized but unripe, either green or turning yellow. The unripe pepper is dried in the sun — mostly on concrete patios (sometimes still on bamboo mats on the ground) — for four to seven days, while the outer flesh is blackened by enzymes and shrinks to the wrinkled skin that contains most of the aromatic power of the spice. A single vine under casual cultivation produces only a pound or two of dried pepper, but a vine under intensive cultivation can yield ten to fifteen pounds. On average, eight thousand to ten thousand black peppercorns make a pound.

White pepper is produced from ripe red berries, washed of the soft, colored outer layer to reveal the smooth whitish core — traditionally by leaving bags of pepper in streams for a week or two. Afterward, the white pepper is dried in the sun. A similar spice is sometimes made nowadays by removing the black coating from black pepper. (In the United States this must be labeled "decorticated black pepper.") The taste is supposed to be slightly stronger than and different from that of true white pepper, which, tasted by itself, has a marked barnyard element. White pepper is, of course, often preferred in light-colored foods, not only in Western cooking but, for instance, in Cantonese. Where color is of no concern, black pepper is better because it is more aromatic. The flavor of white pepper is sometimes considered subtly different, but to me it is just milder and simpler.

For green peppercorns, the berries are harvested green and packed in vinegar or brine, the most flavorful forms, or else freeze-dried or dehydrated. The last method produces a more flavorful peppercorn than the freeze-dried and is preferred in a pepper mill. The spiciness and moderate heat of green peppercorns suggest a less-concentrated version of black pepper (which is, after all, picked at the same unripe stage).

Pink, or red, peppercorns, a novelty introduced during the tumult of nouvelle cuisine, come from *Schinus terebinthifolius*, a plant variously called the Brazilian pepper tree, Christmas berry, or Florida holly. Eating pink peppercorns has caused adverse reactions in some people, and for a time the berries were banned from sale by the FDA. But the French government made a case for the safety of *Schinus terebinthifolius* berries imported from the island of Réunion under the name *baies roses*, "pink berries," and those are again legal. The species, from the size of a large bush to a willowlike tree, is native to Brazil and has become a pest in Florida and, among other places, on Réunion itself. The dried spice is on average slightly larger than a peppercorn, with the red to pink skin dried to a thin brittle shell loosely surrounding a single seed. The flavor is sweet at first, almost citrus, and then somewhat menthol and resinous. The berries have a slight bitterness and little if any heat. Interesting, but odd and not really useful apart from their novelty.

Approximately a dozen related and unrelated plants have been used in various parts of the world as substitutes for black pepper. Some have separate virtues and are really additional seasonings to pepper; not all have a peppery hot bite. One out of the miscellany is melegueta pepper, also called grains of paradise. Today the plant, which belongs to the ginger family, both grows wild and is cultivated; it is used in the cooking and medicine of several West

African countries. The seed was carried across the Sahara to Europe as early as the thirteenth century. Melegueta pepper became an important seasoning, and later the Portuguese brought it by sea from Guinea, then known as the Grain Coast, after the grains of paradise. Elizabeth I is said to have been fond of the spice. Until the practice was outlawed in Britain by George III, it was used to give a false impression of alcoholic strength to beer and liquor. One account compares the aroma to camphor. There are confusing old names, and the various substitutes for melegueta pepper overlap with the half-dozen alternatives to cardamom. So much money was once at stake that substitutes and adulterants were common. (Out of the tangle of spices with similar aromas, in the West only cinnamon and cassia are still prominent. In the United States, either may legally be sold as cinnamon, though cassia is the usual spice.)

Three close relatives to black pepper, once used in the kitchens of the West, are today nearly forgotten by us. One is the cubeb berry (*Piper cubeba*), a drupe from a climbing shrub that is native to Java and now grown in other parts of southeastern Asia and in India. In England in 1307, a pound of cubebs for the "King's Wardrobe" cost nine shillings. Cubebs were used then to season meats and other dishes in a highly spiced, even sugared, Muslim-influenced style that would probably unsettle modern palates. But cubebs have long since fallen out of use.

Despite reading and being assured that I couldn't find cubebs today in the United States, I went looking for them in New York. After several failures I found them in Greenwich Village in the spice shop Aphrodisia. The dried black berry is the size of the largest allspice berries and comes with its stem attached. (It was once called tailed pepper.) Biting into it, I taste tea and a mild muskiness and spice. Ground in a mortar, the berries release an aroma of nutmeg and cumin. Cooking alters the scent to something more currylike, persistent, and still slightly floral, with scarcely a trace of the heat of black pepper.

The second black-pepper relative formerly used in European cooking is Indian long pepper (*P. longum*). Both long and black pepper were found in India by Alexander the Great. The philosopher Theophrastus, pupil of Aristotle along with Alexander, wrote, "Pepper is a fruit, and there are two kinds. One is round ... and it is reddish; the other is elongated and black and has seeds like those of a poppy. And this kind is much stronger than the other." The entire pod of long pepper is used as the spice; it is about an inch and a half long, less than one-quarter inch wide, and slightly tapered. Like black pepper, it is harvested unripe and dried in the sun. For a long period, the Romans valued long pepper more than black.

Julie Sahni, writer and teacher about Indian cooking, kindly sent me a gift of long pepper. She told me it is often possible to find it in Indian markets in America, where I'd looked in vain. I didn't know to ask in the ones that specialize in food from the region of Bombay. (Besides Indian markets, you find unusual spices in some Southeast Asian markets and in shops that sell medicinal herbs in the China-towns of New York and San Francisco, although language can be an almost insurmountable obstacle.) The sweet smell of the ground long pepper gives no warning of the taste. The hot pungency caught me so much off guard it made me laugh. The flavor suggests something of black pepper, wintergreen, cinnamon, and clove. Someone I offered it to compared it to the candies called Red Hots.

The Sanskrit word *pippali* meant "berry" and also "long pepper," and because long pepper was at first the most highly regarded kind of pepper, *pippali* is the root of the word *pepper* in European languages. (Pierre Poivre, eighteenth-century naturalist and administrator of French colonies in the East, spread the planting of pepper, nutmeg, and cinnamon beyond Asia, but he did not give his incredible name to pepper. The French word *poivre* came into the language centuries earlier and is also descended from *pippali*.) The Sanskrit for "black pepper" was *marichi*, which is nearly intact as Indonesian *marieha*.

The third important culinary relative of black pepper is Java long pepper (*P. retrofractum* or alternatively *P. officinarum*), once exported by the Dutch. It grows wild in Java, but most is cultivated by small farmers. I've never found it to taste it. An Indonesian pepper exporter told me that Java long pepper used to be imported into the United States but no more. He said the Indonesian word is *cabe merah* (cha-BAY may-RAH, with a rolled r), the first word of which means "pepper." It may still be exported to Singapore, spice-trading capital of the East before the days of telexes and faxes. Java long pepper, like Indian long pepper, is used as seasoning and as medicine in various parts of southern Asia. A friend who lives in Indonesia and is served by an "ancient and feisty cook," Ibu Tini, shed further light. "Yes," he wrote, "there is a pepper called *Piper retrofractum* grown in central Java, but the USDA will not let me ship you any samples. A friend did find some at the Bogor Botanical Gardens (apparently, these peppers are not that common or preferred). I was going to try them and tell you how they tasted but they were put in the refrigerator (without any special instructions) and the next morning they were gone! The night watchman said they were delicious but not as hot as the small red peppers, which he prefers."

Having tasted cubebs and Indian long pepper, I begin to see black pepper as merely a single possibility among several: one may speak of peppers. In that light, it may be easier to understand the orchestration of spice flavors in various Asian cuisines. The variety of spices today unknown to Americans and Europeans also suggests a question: How inevitable was our final selection of spices?

It is often said that in the Middle Ages pepper and other spices were used to disguise the taste of bad meat ("the most repulsive fare," says one writer). Maybe. Meat was more important in the medieval diet than in today's, but much meat was well preserved by salt. If so, how much bad meat can really have been eaten? Marginally bad meat was probably more acceptable then than it is to us, but those who could afford pepper could certainly afford to reject tainted meat. And those who couldn't afford spices ate little fresh meat of any quality.

It seems more convincing that pepper and other spices were valued for their prestige, exoticism, supposed physical powers (at a time when food wasn't distinguished from medicine), and for the variety they gave to a dull diet. The medieval table was without potatoes, tomatoes, corn, chocolate, tea, coffee, vanilla, allspice, and the choice of vegetables was altogether limited compared to ours. The first lemons and bitter oranges, along with sugar and spices, were likely brought back to Europe by returning Crusaders. Perhaps spices distracted from the gamy taste of even the domesticated meat of the time. And like rich clothing and other displays of opulence, the manner of eating must have served partly to put the populace in awe. The nobility's practice of gilding food with saffron must have been not only exciting but socially distinguishing. Lacking pepper, even the poor might gather sour herbs and obtain pungent heat from cress, nasturtium, horseradish (in Eastern Europe), and mustard. There were also aromatic sweet herbs to be had, at least from certain gardens.

The early trading wealth of Venice (whose government was expressly a mechanism to serve commerce and whose palaces were also warehouses) came from salt, which was originally gathered in the surrounding marshes. From its beginning with salt, the city-state of Venice by the tenth century had pacified and gained control of the Adriatic. Construing the Crusades as an opportunity for profit, Venice contracted to supply its fleets for transporting knights and pilgrims and profited handsomely, as well as gaining territory and trading rights in the newly opened lands. After the Crusades had reawakened European interest in the spices and goods of the East, the greatest naval and trading powers of the Mediterranean were Venice and Genoa, rivals until Venice became dominant in the 1400s. Venetian merchants bought their spices from the Arab middlemen in Egypt and the Levant. The city's reputation, like that of pepper, became part of the substance of its power. Without Italian wealth from trade, there might have been no Renaissance.

Like other spices, peppercorns were valuable because they were small, easily transported, and lasted indefinitely at normal temperatures. Pepper was so concentrated a form of value that it was used as money. For five centuries scarcity kept the price high, until the Portuguese rounded the tip of Africa and found an all-sea route to India and Indonesia, avoiding reliance on Arab and Italian merchants.

Even today, the names of the kinds of black pepper in commerce are richly exotic to Western ears. They are place-names signifying where pepper is grown or the ports from which it is shipped. From India, Malabar (formerly Alleppey, a port on the Malabar Coast) and Tellicherry (port); from Indonesia, Lampong (province of Sumatra); from Malaysia, Sarawak (where pepper is the main crop). Among kinds of white pepper, the best known and perhaps the best is Muntok (named for a now-obscure port on the Indonesian island of Bangka). Besides these places, smaller amounts of pepper are grown in Sri Lanka, Madagascar, Thailand, Cambodia, Vietnam, China, and in Africa and Central America. Pepper also comes from Brazil, which is today a major producer, although its whole peppercorns rarely find their way to the US retail market.

Tellicherry nowadays refers not to the product of that region but to a grade of Indian peppercorns — the largest ones. Tellicherry is distinctly more pungent and aromatic than almost any other pepper. Much of it goes to Italy for *salame*. An oil distilled from Tellicherry pepper is more intense; some of it is used in perfume. The differences in the flavors of black pepper from various parts of the world result mainly from the variety of black pepper that is grown in a place and from the stage at which it is picked (and to a lesser extent from where and how it is grown). At a certain point of green unripeness, reached at about four and a half to five months, flavor is the most concentrated, after which it declines. Chinese and Brazilian peppers are supposed to be milder than others; the Chinese may prefer milder pepper.

Why pepper? Why was it the most expensive, the favorite seasoning of Europe before all others, the one that drove explorers across oceans? The answers may be more obvious than it at first appears. Lacking the narrowly defined personalities of most other important spices, pepper enhances and at the same time is submissive. It blends easily with meat, fish, and vegetables in a way that suits the temper of the West. Pepper's heat teases gently, hardly at all. It burns only when used in such quantity that its aromatic component becomes ludicrously overpowering — unlike the searing capsicums with their comparatively neutral aroma. Pepper is a flatterer that insinuates itself into dissimilar foods from roast beef to fish, eggs, soup, green beans, salad, pfeffernüsse. The aroma of freshly ground pepper heightens even the most well-prepared dishes. Only vanilla, in sweet dishes, performs at all similarly. Pepper can appear in dish after dish without cloying or tiring the senses.

Besides its broad swathe of applications, black pepper has a specific affinity for cured meats, primarily the rich tastes of cured beef and pork. And pepper belongs in any meat pâté or terrine, often as part of the variable mixture called *quatre épices*. Pepper nearly always forms a part of marinades. It complements fresh cheeses such as mozzarella, and it goes well with raw bulb fennel (thinly sliced and dressed with lemon, oil, and salt). I habitually put coarse pepper into pizza dough. Less obviously, pepper, like other spices, flatters fruit: melon, strawberries, peaches, pears. But pepper almost never plays a leading role in any dish (some exceptions are steak au poivre, *sauce poivrade* for game, and scrapple).

Richard Olney, a careful writer about food and a demanding cook, bars pepper from any long-cooked liquid preparation such as a braise or stock. He finds the aroma disappears and the pepper turns bitter. I understand him to mean that the caramelizing (browning) that occurs during grilling, roasting, or frying hides the bitterness, while in a liquid it is exposed. The hot principal in pepper is piperine, an alkaloid, which by itself is certainly acrid and bitter. Out of curiosity, I've experimented with cooking exaggerated amounts of pepper in liquids, but I haven't perceived a problem. (Possibly I am less sensitive to bitterness, perceiving it here only as a note of complexity.) I often put the whole corns into rich liquids along with a few allspice berries or a clove or two, and sometimes cubebs. The spicing is easily overdone and in most preparations should be all but imperceptible.

Some cooks make their own pepper mixtures, usually of some ratio of black to white pepper together with a seventh or eighth part of broken-up allspice — sometimes with green peppercorns and even pink ones. I've tried these, but my inclinations are conservative. I don't think that white or green add much, and pink is off the subject. For some uses, I like eight parts of black peppercorns to one part of cracked allspice. (Lacking a small mortar, the allspice berries can be adequately crushed under the back of a wooden spoon.) You lose valuable perfume by breaking the spice in advance, but there is no other way to spread the nuance evenly through the mix.

The most pleasing aromatic qualities of pepper are the most fleeting. Pepper must be ground fresh. Through happenstance I had ended up with four mills, then, giving in to my urge for a more complete selection of possibilities, I bought a fifth. Each of these mills produces a somewhat different grind. Two (a coarse and a medium) contain Tellicherry pepper, two hold Tellicherry pepper tinged with allspice, and one contains Muntok white pepper. Just as salt should be on the table for those whose taste calls for more of it, so a pepper mill should always be on the table.

8

An Aged Country Ham

The most exquisite peak in culinary art is conquered when you do right by a ham, for a ham, in the very nature of the process it has undergone since it last stalked on its own feet, combines in its flavor the tang of smoky autumnal woods, the maternal softness of earthy fields delivered of their crop children, the wineyness of a late sun, the intimate kiss of fertilizing rain, and the bite of fire. You must slice it thin, too, almost as thin as this page you have in your hands. The making of a ham dinner, like the making of a gentleman, starts a long, long time before the event.

— W. B. COURTNEY

An aged Southern country ham, unless it has been rubbed clean for commerce, appears as a nearly Paleolithic object to those who have seldom or never encountered one. The ham is old. Farmers who cure their own hams wait at least nine months before eating them; some devotees delay for two years. The ham is a hind leg, cut long on the hock and high toward the loin. It may measure two feet from end to end, and it weighs from one to two dozen pounds. The rind is an uncertain smoke brown (though in a few areas of the South hams are not smoked); the exposed lean is often coated with a fine grit of black pepper over which is a harmless growth of green mold. The mold is a sign of authenticity. Without it, a ham may not have the rarefied tang that connoisseurs seek. The outside of the raw ham is only modestly redolent of smoke, pepper,

75

and hog — compared with the intensity within. Raw or cooked, the ham is much saltier than any brined ham. The latter is all that survives in New England or has ever been made in most areas of the country. The usual brined ham is so bland that it must be refrigerated or it will spoil. Some country hams are made to be saltier and drier than others. Aging further dries a ham, concentrating both salt and flavor. The salt is too strong for a desalinated palate, but, once you get past the salt, the flavor spoils you for any lesser sort of ham.

The making of a ham, like the making of other foods, was once perforce tied to the seasons. On Southern farms and at certain Southern packing houses, the most traditional hams are still put down only in the fall and aged at prevailing outdoor temperatures. Long ago, curing hams was not an unusual skill. "That's just something that went along with living," says a current practitioner whose ancestors arrived in Virginia in the mid-1600s.

The qualities of a ham, like those of other foods, reflected the practices and resources of the place where it was made: the common breed of pig, its diet, age, the way the ham was cured, the available salt. The name of a ham is usually the name of a place. Even today famous names are Parma, Bayonne, Westphalian, Smithfield, York, and Paris. The last two are mild and brined and long since detached from a place of origin ("Paris" never really meant more than a city-style ham), and all the names probably signify less than they once did.

In Old World or New, pigs, like cattle, were slaughtered after the harvest during a late fall spell of cold weather, so the meat wouldn't spoil before the salt penetrated to the bone. After the killing, the perishable offal was eaten immediately along with some fresh meat, a rare treat for those without access to the butcher shops of towns. Part of this small wealth might be shared among neighbors. But most of the hog was salted or pickled in brine, or salted and dried in the form of sausage. In some places, the meat was salted, cooked in fat, and preserved from the air in the same fat (potted, as in French *confit*). The slaughter was also a way to cull lesser animals, since a farm family could afford to feed only the best through the winter.

And in various places hams were made of other meats than pork — wild boar, beef, mutton.

It is possible to overstate the old local influences, and Dorothy Hartley in *Food in England* (1954) may give too much credit to former ways (she gives none at all to the influx of fat Chinese pigs that produced the rotund nineteenth-century breeds, and she jumbles her pork nomenclature), but: "In the [old] pictures you see the varied characters of the orchard pig, the moorland pig, the wheat-land pig, and the forager pig. These pigs had character before they were pork. Thus we get the Wiltshire bacon, the York ham, the Devon and Somerset bacons, the Suffolk flitch, the Norfolk, the Lancashire, and Durham bacons. All these pigs had some definite *reason* for their diversity." (*Bacon* is an unspecific word that can refer to the whole cured side of a pig.)

From the Middle Ages until the intensive breeding work of the nineteenth century, races of pigs were lean and some looked very like wild boars. All were leaner even than the hogs that toward the end of the twentieth century were bred away from the lard hog (developed well before there was cheap vegetable oil for cooking) to meet the demand for less-fatty meat. American Southerners who cure hams today don't claim to detect much difference among hams from the various current breeds. And instead of raising their own, many farmers buy the fresh hams they use for curing. Most prefer a moderate degree of fat, and the fat is delicious. But the more interesting flavor transformation takes place in the lean (which is why one wants bacon or salt pork with a good streak of lean).

The intensity of pork flavor in a ham depends largely on the pig's diet. The pig is a highly economical producer of meat, if, instead of being fed grain, it is allowed to forage for its food in pastures or woods. Pasture, meaning mostly grasses, produces stronger-tasting pork, as does a woodland diet of acorns, beechnuts, bark, roots, and nearly anything a pig can reach or root up. Roving pigs tended long ago by a swineherd, or more recently, and occasionally still, let loose in Southern woods, ate this way. In the South, they were penned and fed grain to fatten them before killing. An ancient European practice was to knock down acorns for the pigs in the fall. It isn't hard to see the link between these nuts and the peanuts that used to be fed to hogs in peanut-growing areas of the South.

The curing method has the most influence on the taste of the ham, assuming the beast is reasonably well fed and young. (Today, hogs are killed at about 235 pounds and six to eight months old.) To cure meat is to treat it with salt in order to preserve it. A standard old formula is ten pounds of salt per hundredweight of meat. But some traditional hams are cured with less, and I've been told that Virginia farmers often used twice that standard. Besides salt, the cure may contain saltpeter (potassium nitrate, or nowadays in its place sodium nitrate or nitrite). Saltpeter is an antioxidant that reduces the danger of botulism. It has been used for centuries, at first inadvertently, since it is a natural contaminant of some deposits of salt. Very little is required to be effective, although some old cures call for a dangerous amount of it. Saltpeter slightly changes the flavor (improves it, according to some tastes), and it fixes the deep mahogany red of raw ham, which later pales somewhat in cooking. Neither saltpeter nor its chemical relatives are necessary. But if they aren't used, the USDA requires additional salt, and the color will be a duller red.

The mixture for the cure sometimes includes sugar or a "secret" ingredient. The salt mixture is rubbed into the ham, with special care taken over the parts not covered by skin. Afterward, a further heavy layer of white salt is scattered over the ham. Usually, the salt is put on in two applications, the second five to ten days after the first. And if the salt melts as it draws out the meat's moisture, especially during humid weather, more is sprinkled on. Curing lasts from thirty to fifty days, depending on the size of the ham. Afterward the salt is given a period to "equalize" throughout the meat, before the ham is smoked. Smoke is another antioxidant that helps in preservation.

Long, long ago in Europe, hams may have been smoked not by

intention but by the happenstance that fires were lit regularly in the fall. Many fireplaces were less than aerodynamically sound, and some of their smoke was released into the kitchen. Karen Hess, critic and culinary historian, says, "In northern climes smoking would have gone on almost serendipitously — that is, hams, sausages, etc., were hung from the rafters; you see this in remote parts of France even yet." Usually, meats were smoked high up in the huge old cooking fireplaces, poor at heating and backbreaking to cook in, but sources of the ideal range of degrees and kinds of heat for all the operations of cooking except baking. During smoking, a ham is carefully kept from growing too warm. It shouldn't weep fat, and it must remain raw.

The refinements that occur during the months that follow produce the fine, faint flavors of an aged ham. The changes are accomplished by enzymes and myriad small reactions that occur within the meat. The ham typically loses 20 to 25 percent of its weight; farm hams usually lose more. The USDA requires that a country ham lose 18 percent of its weight and reach 4 percent salt — so it won't spoil outside refrigeration. Some producers aim just above the 4 percent minimum, but most hams contain 5 to 6 and even 7 percent salt. A long hock protects at least one end from excessive drying. The USDA also says that the processing must follow a schedule of times and temperatures. The combined salt, dryness, and aging eliminate possible trichinae, which scarcely any American pork carries anyway. A lesser country ham can be marketed after only sixty to seventy days. A sign of quality in the meat of year-old hams with exceptional flavor is white dots here and there, the size of grains of salt; the same substance, formed by the breakdown of protein, occurs in certain well-aged cheeses.

The American South is a huge and varied area, but there is only a little evidence of regional styles of ham within it. Individual farmers do cure ham in distinct styles, but asking a farmer about regional differences is probably the wrong tactic. He may have no experience

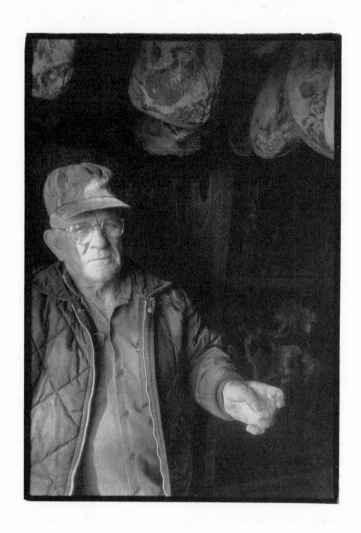

Tiny Guier, farmer and champion ham-curer,
in his smokehouse. Trigg County, Kentucky, 1997.

of hams from outside his area. Anyway, no one off the farm that I've spoken to claims that you can tell by taste that a ham was cured in Virginia or Kentucky or Tennessee or anywhere else. However, you might risk the generalization that Virginia hams tend to be saltier than some. And apparently mountain folk are less likely to smoke their hams than are people who live in more humid coastal areas, where the heat of a fire may once have speeded drying.

The local traditions that dominated in Europe were shuffled together in America, and neighbors often took divergent approaches. The Georgia mountaineers described in *The Foxfire Book* frequently salted down their meat while it was still warm after the killing. The salt was sometimes mixed with molasses and black and red pepper. Some people weighed the meat and measured the salt and some didn't. The ratio varied from five pounds of salt for two hundred pounds of meat to ten pounds of salt for one hundred pounds of meat. Some smokehouses had cracks to let out the smoke, and others were sealed against insects. Some people who smoked their meat used hickory; others, oak; and, a few people, corncobs. Smoking lasted from two to six days. For aging, one man would coat his ham with mixed brown sugar, red pepper, and saltpeter and seal it in a box. A woman surrounded hers with a bushel of corn in a box. A man surrounded his with ashes, and his grandmother used cornmeal.

During aging, especially in the South, larvae-laying insects were a common problem, particularly the flies called skippers. In hope of defeating them, pepper, black or red or a mix, was rubbed into the part of the ham not protected by skin. Insects can't get at the hams in today's commercial smokehouses, but a black-pepper coating is still used in a bow to tradition. By the time pepper is added, the ham is too dry for its flavor to penetrate much below the surface. Similarly, smoke doesn't enter deep into the ham. To protect the hams further, often they were sewn in the cloth bags that are still common. Hams must be aged in a dry place, usually the smokehouse. A Southern country ham can be eaten young, but a lot of people wouldn't give you a nickel for a young ham.

Some brine curing was practiced here and there in the South, but in a warm climate brine tends to spoil, as it can during hot weather in the most northern states. Occasionally, a family that used a brine cure would lose all its hams. Southerners preferred the dry cure because it was more reliable, although back in England some brine cures are followed by drying and aging, with excellent results.

A brined ham (except those English ones later dried and aged) never approaches the flavor of a dry-cured ham. Traditional pickles, as the brines are often called, contained herbs and spices, such as bay leaves, juniper berries, peppercorns, nutmeg, thyme, and cloves, and often sugar. The complex savor of an aged dry-cured ham would only be compromised if herbs and spices were introduced to it. (Actually, most American hams are not only brined but injected with brine, so they contain about 10 percent added water.) Dr. Robert Kelly, retired professor at Virginia Polytechnic Institute, who judged hams for many years, said to me of brined hams, "There's nothing wrong with them," but, "personally, I don't like them. I don't think they have very much flavor." The pickled ham is moister and tastes more like roasted fresh pork than it does country ham. Dry-cured ham makes no pretensions to matching the qualities of fresh meat. It transcends mere juiciness to arrive at a finer state.

Hams were exported from the small Virginia town of Smithfield as long ago as the eighteenth century. Myth attributes the original curing method to the Indians, and the Indians did dry strips of venison and probably other meats on a wooden frame over a fire. But they didn't have sufficient salt to cure hams. Robert Beverley wrote in *The History of Virginia* in 1722, "They have no Salt among them, but for seasoning use the Ashes of Hiccory, Stickwood, or some other Wood or Plant, affording a Salt Ash." Pigs arrived only with the English colonists, and American cures, dry or brine, were the traditional English ones. The smoking credited to the Indians was and is typically English and less common on the Continent.

The original Virginia "ham law" of 1926 declared that genuine Smithfield-cured pork must be "cut from the carcasses of peanut-fed hogs, raised in the peanut belt of the State of Virginia or the State of North Carolina," and processed in the town of Smithfield. The fame of Smithfield was tied to peanuts. Hogs used to be put in the peanut fields to glean them after the harvest, but apparently the harvest became too thorough. The law was rewritten in the 1960s to eliminate mention of peanuts, and today peanut-fed hogs are rare, if not nonexistent. Hogs for Smithfield hams are typically fed corn and soybeans, and they may be raised anywhere in the country. The old peanut-fed hams are remembered as having softer, yellower fat and oilier meat, and they didn't dry out as fast as other hams. Peanut-fed pork was popular only in the South; elsewhere, hogs with yellow fat brought a lower price. But there are surely old-timers in Virginia who believe that the only way to cure a ham is to start with a peanut-fed hog.

Now the only requirements for a Smithfield ham are that it be processed within Smithfield by dry salting and aged for at least six months. So unless there is something in the air around Smithfield, as Parmesans believe there is around Parma (specifically, around the town of Langhirano, south of the city), there is nothing especially characteristic of Smithfield hams. Anyway, most of the extraordinary number of hams processed in the town aren't "genuine Smithfield" under the law and don't receive that label. They are marketed in the reflected glory of the name by the three huge Smithfield packers. And even the label "genuine" is no guarantee of flavor. On the published recommendation of a respected cook, one January I ordered Gwaltney's Genuine Smithfield ham, supposedly the best of the surviving true Smithfield hams. When I served it, the Gwaltney was roundly condemned as "one-dimensional." I discovered that the company had sold out of fully aged hams at Christmastime; this one was only six to seven months old — aged at ambient temperatures at the wrong time of year.

Other and perhaps better packing houses are located outside Smithfield. S. Wallace Edwards and Sons is located in Surry,

Virginia. As Sam Edwards recounts, the business began in the 1920s when his great-grandfather operated the Jamestown-Surry ferry. His grandfather had the idea of selling ham sandwiches to the ferry passengers. Within a few years, sandwiches led to whole hams and whole hams led to a packing house. The ham produced today by the original Edwards cure is called Wigwam Brand. Country ham used to be a household staple, but currently Edwards sells a hundred of its mild hams for every Wigwam; thirty years ago they sold more Wigwams. Sam Edwards explains that "everyone had a country ham in their refrigerator 365 days a year." Today's Wigwam buyers are likely to be "into food," and thanks to them, sales of the Wigwam are holding steady. The interest in regional foods helps. Some Southern restaurants serve the ham raw as they would prosciutto.

The Wigwam is near the lower limit of country-ham saltiness. Each fall, the traditional hams are held initially at low temperatures by refrigeration (no waiting for a natural cold spell) until the cure penetrates. Then they are transferred to an old smokehouse reserved just for them. When the smokehouse is full, that's it for the year. The hams are smoked with hickory and aged for at least ten months. Each ham matures at its own pace. Like other country hams, before they are sold, the Wigwams are checked with a probe like an ice pick that reaches the bone. Appearance, feel, and the aroma at the surface and on the probe together tell when the ham is ready for the market.

The Pruden Packing Company in Suffolk, Virginia, started in 1917, makes a traditional ham in a drier, saltier style (which a few people find not salty enough). R.A. Howell, general manager of the business, quotes the current Mr. Pruden: "If something's not broke, don't fix it." The oldest smokehouse is reserved for the old-fashioned hams. Fires are lit in the basement and wet sawdust, mostly oak and sometimes hickory, is added to create the smoke. R.A. Howell says another packing house nearby uses exactly the same cure, but some small difference in the way it is carried out results in a consistent difference you can taste. When he was growing up, his family joined with their neighbors every fall to kill and process about twenty-five hogs. I asked him about the importance of a hog's diet to the taste of a ham and was told that although there are people with definite opinions about feed, "I've never seen nobody get up from the table yet." Old-time Virginians feel "you've got to have a country ham to season with. That's just the way they think."

I know of no reason why the finest country ham cannot be produced on a fairly large scale in a packing house, but many Southerners prefer to buy their hams directly from individual farmers, who may cure only two dozen hams each fall. These farmers often attribute the flavor of their hams to the summer "sweats," although some larger operations would describe the loss of fat as "dripping money." John Taylor of Charleston, a historian of the low-country food of South Carolina, says, "The best hams that I have ever eaten were from very small farms in the western part of Tennessee and middle Kentucky." Those are areas he knows well; not that equally good hams aren't made elsewhere. Of a certain South Carolina farmer's ham Taylor says, "It's just incredible. It'll drive you crazy." Yet ham makes little appearance in historical Southern cookbooks. Taylor says, "*Of course* — they take it for granted." Now that the South has lost many of its farms, and now that fewer of the farmers who remain cure their own hams, conscious appreciation has taken hold. "The connoisseurship came with nostalgia. Everybody I know who has roots in South Carolina that are deep talks about the smokehouse."

Even in its partial decline, the tradition of country ham is vital enough that country ham is likely to appear on a Southern table at any meal with grits or biscuits, or with fancier accompaniments. One area that produces outstanding country hams is Trigg County, Kentucky, in the western part of the state. Cadiz (KAY-deez) is the county seat and site of a well-known ham festival. Douglas Freeman, whose ham won first place at the festival a few years back, owns a small farm outside town where he raises hogs, cattle, and tobacco. About his cure he says, "I've sort of got a little secret." But the cure includes salt, saltpeter, and sugar. "I bury 'em in this cure for approximately three weeks, depending on what size they are." The hams are smoked with hickory sawdust and sassafras. And during the summer inside the smokehouse, it gets "just pretty warm so the grease will drip out of 'em. That's how I think they get their flavor, going through the summer." The hams lose 30 percent of their weight from start to finish.

Twice when I've tried to order an old-style country ham by phone from a packing house that also made a milder ham, the ham I asked for was disparaged to me as salty. With severe warnings about the old-style ham, the telephone voice steered me firmly toward the milder one, until I nearly had to argue. Accent or place of origin must function as a kind of password, since a Southern friend to whom I described this had never heard of such a thing. Apparently, uninitiated customers have complained about genuine country ham.

The proper old product doesn't come cheap, although it is much less expensive than the famous imported hams. Once purchased, it can be stored in a cool, dry place, well protected from insects, until it is about two years old, but not much longer, because eventually it really will become too dry and salty.

When you "boil" a whole country ham, you have to spend a day in or near the kitchen. The actual technique is not boiling, which dries and toughens a ham, but gentle poaching in water that doesn't reach a bubble. An enormous pot is needed. The task is unlike the sort of cooking most people do these days, and a number of people consider it a messy, unpleasant chore, although poaching a ham isn't something anyone does more than once or twice a year. Instead some people recommend buying precooked country hams, which are commonly sold by Southern packers. They may cook the ham as carefully as you would at home. I don't know because I haven't fooled around with precooked hams. I enjoy the whole experience of a ham, starting with scrubbing it.

With a stiff brush and a stream of water, you clean off mold, excess pepper, and other surface matter. Most people then soak the ham to reintroduce some moisture to the dry exterior before cooking starts and, according to the popular theory, to remove salt. The saltiness of the ham and your taste for salt are supposed to determine the length of the soaking — from overnight up to several days. One thinks of salt cod, where it is possible to soak out nearly all the salt and all the flavor. But the texture of a ham is much more resistant than that of a fish. You can soak a country ham for forty-eight hours and perceive hardly a trace of salt in the soaking water, which will, however, taste of smoke. Changing the water once or twice, as some do, is futile. In any case, most of the ham is covered by rind and thick fat, so the water has limited access to the meat. But soaking may give a head start to the slight rehydration that occurs during cooking. Karen Hess believes that if some water is not reintroduced to the dry meat fibers, they will only become tough and stringy in cooking. John Taylor says, "It is just done. Who am I to question the wisdom of so many people who have gone before me?"

What is certainly essential to the flavor, texture, and moisture of the ham is gentle cooking. I haven't sacrificed any hams to novel experiments, and I can't swear to what goes on inside the ham during cooking. But probably the ham loses a little of its modest residue of moisture initially and later takes some back on, just as liquid reenters meat during the latter part of careful braising. Most of the movement of moisture inside the ham certainly takes place near the surface. And that's just as well, since the outside, especially the part protected by rind and fat, is harder, drier, and saltier than the inside. After cooking, the outermost meat has lost much of its taste. If you cook a ham for too many hours, you lose altogether too much salt and flavor to the cooking water.

Many people add bay leaves and spices to the water, or cook the ham in cider, cola, or some liquid other than water, but I question how much the flavors of those liquids penetrate the ham. And certainly those flavors only obscure the taste of a special ham. With a mild brined or young ham, however, it makes sense to put wine, fresh or hard cider, spices, or other flavorings into the liquid. A French addition to the pot is a bed of fragrant hay.

The ham is raised slowly to poaching temperature, about 180 degrees Fahrenheit, over two hours, and it is cooked for roughly five to seven hours. The time needed reflects the length, width, and greatest thickness, but devising a precise formula for the irregular shape is difficult. My rule of thumb is: five and a half to six hours at 175 to 180 degrees for a fifteen-pound ham; add or subtract twenty minutes for each pound above or below fifteen. This works partly because slow initial heating and gradual final cooling provide a forgiving leeway; the ham is left in its pot of hot liquid to cool overnight. Some people wrap the pot in an old quilt or blanket so that the ham cools even more slowly. The cooling period may be the time when the ham reabsorbs liquid.

The next day, the cook removes all the discolored surface meat and the rind, creating a remarkable amount of waste and exposing the fat. The fat is trimmed to an even layer of a quarter to half an inch. A wide border of fat is handsome on a slice, and the individual can decide how much of it to eat. During cooking, the thick exterior fat doesn't enter the lean. And only occasionally is a slice visibly marbled with fat.

For a more formal presentation, and for the pleasure of eating warm ham, the bare fat is glazed or covered with bread crumbs and browned. Before the days of iron and steel ovens, this was accomplished by roasting before an open fire. Mary Randolph's recipe "To Toast a Ham" in *The Virginia House-wife* gives the idea, although in 1824 she already mentions an oven, but perhaps this is merely a reflective metal oven for setting before the fire. In the old fashion, she covers the fat not with sugar but with bread crumbs. Karen Hess says, "Those South Carolinians who are traditional *still* eschew sweetness until the dessert course, and make quite a point of it."

When people speak of baking a ham, they often mean glazing or toasting an already poached ham, but you can bake or roast a previously uncooked ham, if it is not too aged. Assuming hog killing in the fall, this is the kind of ham you would have the following spring at Easter. Before baking, the ham is trimmed of surface fat and lean;

and it is baked in a medium oven for three to four hours. (I haven't done this, but the ham should reach a temperature of 145 degrees Fahrenheit throughout.) Such a ham would benefit from frequent basting, as was sometimes done in the past with a mixture of water and cider vinegar.

But why cook the ham at all? It is safe to eat as it is, if it has been salted and aged as prescribed by the USDA. And the raw ham is deliciously close kin to prosciutto (albeit the Parma ham isn't smoked — but then, the smoke flavor is slight inside a country ham). Until the present, serving raw ham was unheard of in the South, although children would sometimes pull off a piece of raw ham in the smokehouse to gnaw on. (And they might get into trouble because the violated ham could spoil.) But in continental Europe, hams that are dry-cured just as carefully are not cooked — not whole, anyway. The explanation for the American preference for the taste and texture of cooked ham must be cultural, although fear of trichinosis may play a role. Like our cures, our habits in eating ham were originally British, and historically the British didn't eat their hams raw. But the earliest origins of the preference for cooked ham may be lost to time.

The popular everyday way to cook ham in the South is to fry it. Quarter-inch-thick steaks or very thin slices of raw ham are cooked briefly, so as not to be made tough, and served with red-eye gravy, which is made simply by rinsing the pan with coffee or water and pouring the juices over the meat. Of course, the ham is accompanied by biscuits or grits or some other starch to offset its intensity. The driest hams are appropriate for poaching, not frying. Many people keep an aged raw ham in the refrigerator, or merely a cool place, and cut meat from it as needed over a period of weeks, although the outer slice will dry and it will discolor if exposed to light. (Some specialists warn that a cut ham, whether raw or cooked, is vulnerable to spoilage after only one or two weeks of refrigeration.) Ham is often frozen, and it suffers less from freezing than most meats do.

Those unused to the salt of country ham will probably understand it best as a condiment, served alongside another meat, such as a roast bird, or as one of a selection of meats. That is the way ham was and often is served at large dinners. A flavor has very different effects depending on its intensity. Like subtle notes in perfume that disappear when it is spilled, the thin slices of ham reveal flavors that are concealed in the intensity of a thick piece.

The whole ham is ideal for a buffet or other large gathering. (Less than a whole ham can't be cooked properly.) But if there is no large gathering, what to do with a poached whole ham? Ham keeps, in my experience, for several weeks or longer. Refrigeration reduces the opportunities for mold on a moist ham, which shouldn't be wrapped too closely. Slices are taken as needed to make a snack or a meal and to flavor innumerable dishes. Finely diced ham goes into the *soffritto* or *mirepoix* that begins many preparations. And ham goes into pasta dishes, egg dishes, braises, many sauces, sausages, and terrines. The ham becomes tender if it is cooked only briefly in liquid. Beware that a little strong ham goes a long way. Ultimately, the bones flavor beans and soup; some people hold that the bones are the real point of the ham. In any case, there is no need to do anything more complicated with the meat than eat thin slices between bread. It must have been a deracinated city-dweller who defined eternity as two people and a ham. Raw or cooked, a ham was generally always on hand in the past and it isn't rare today.

Few American foods are both made as well as they possibly can be and have a long, continuous history of quality. What a pleasure to know one of them. An aged Southern country ham is equal to any of the world's great hams.

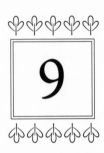

9

Bay Leaves

Cooks are frequently told to use imported European bay leaves — not the California ones. As Julia Child et al. gently advise in *Mastering the Art of French Cooking*, "American bay is stronger and a bit different in taste than European bay. We suggest you buy imported leaves." In appearance, the dried leaves cannot be mistaken for one another. The California leaf is longer and has turned a deep green that is quite distinct from the light, dull gray-green of the European. The aroma of American *Umbellularia californica* is powerful; European *Laurus nobilis* is, by comparison, subtle and submissive.

The two laurels do inhabit similar environments. The European is indigenous to the Mediterranean basin, and California laurel is native to that large part of California with a Mediterranean climate. The growing plants are much alike, both evergreen, both characteristic of the Mediterranean-type mix of trees and shrubs that in California is called chaparral. European bay laurel grows especially near the coasts of the three continents surrounding the Mediterranean. It is often found near streams. But the range of the plant extends inland as well as northeast to the Black Sea coast of Turkey. Usually, it is a shrub or small tree, although in favorable conditions it struggles to a height of sixty feet. European bay will also grow outside its native habitat, as it does in many parts of California. Unlike the ash-hued dry leaves, the living leaves are dark green and somewhat glossy, as leathery and as thin as the dried. The plants are slow growing, with dense foliage, especially when clipped. Bay laurel is used as seasoning in all the countries where it is found.

A jar full of dried European bay has little scent, but a freshly dried batch of California bay I once had smelled rudely to me of bay plus particularly rank rocket (arugula) and bold nutmeg. A few weeks later it had subsided to nutmeg alone, distinct enough to recall eggnog. Rubbing the leaves opens the microscopic oil glands and releases much more odor, the simple way to judge quality. When rubbed, California leaves produce a camphor-and-paint smell irritating to the nose, and their taste is awful. The leaf leaves a menthol-like sting in the mouth. Both kinds are peppery, but there they diverge.

One spice wholesaler calls the substitution of California for European bay leaves "preposterous," denouncing the California species as "paintlike, chemical." Strange to think of cooking with it, though incredibly some spice companies push it, and California Indians did perhaps flavor with it. To be more blunt than Julia Child, California bay is unimaginable as a substitute for European bay.

Few of the various plants called laurel are related, but they are vaguely alike in evergreen appearance, generally aromatic, and more or less poisonous. The mountain laurel of eastern North America is dangerous to livestock, the seeds have poisoned birds, and honey from the flowers is toxic to eat. Oleander is especially deadly. And the bitter-almond scent of cherry laurel, common in Britain, derives from prussic acid, close in toxicity and composition to cyanide. The great Victorian cook Mrs. Beeton wrote, "It ought to be known, that there are two kinds of bay-trees, — the Classic laurel, whose leaves are comparatively harmless, and the Cherry-laurel, which is the one whose leaves are employed in ... blanc-mange, puddings, custards, etc.; but, when acted upon by water, they develop prussic acid, and, therefore, but a small number of the leaves should be used at a time." Probably none at all. Bay rum, the old-fashioned hair tonic and aftershave lotion, has been known to irritate the skin. It was originally made by distilling the leaves of the West Indian bay-rum tree in rum. California bay contains minor quantities of yet another toxin. And even European bay laurel is narcotic or sedative in sufficient quantity.

A tip of the dried leaf of European bay tastes piney and has a gratifying perfume. It is both bitter and pleasantly aromatic. Besides its obvious components of nutmeg and pepper, it has been called pungent, balsamic, spicy, oily-resinous, and — perhaps reaching — compared to vanilla, delicate lemon, and clove. It is also known as sweet bay, and its ambiguous qualities can be interpreted as either savory or sweet.

Straddling the distinction, tomatoes are clearly enhanced by bay. Most savory combinations are similarly familiar. In sweet combinations, bay's bitterness is probably best suited to wild fruit or the concentrated taste of dried fruit. Bitterness is often a component of wildness, and in any case strong flavors balance bitterness. A leaf added to dried figs cooked in wine is excellent. (Soak a dozen figs — or prunes — overnight in a half cup of white wine; then gently simmer liquid, fruit, two tablespoons of honey, and a small bay leaf for about twenty minutes in a covered pan.) With more delicate sweets, an unpleasant bitterness can show baldly. Further, pears cooked in *red* wine with bay and spices tend to have a medicinal taste resulting from the simultaneous bitter, herbal, and sweet.

Bay's bitterness is more lasting than its aromatic presence. The cook's defense is to employ freshly dried leaves. Brown are certainly inferior. I cannot decide whether small leaves are truly sweeter, as some believe. Dried bay, unlike dried basil or chervil, is close to the fresh herb. Yet fresh leaves from the plants in my window are sweeter than any dried, sweet in the sense that cinnamon and clove are sweet. And they have a grassy freshness. Patience Gray writes in *Honey from a Weed*, "In the Salento it grows wild in the shelter of ravines. It was by transplanting one of these into the garden that the conviction dawned that it should be used fresh not dried." Besides her more conventional uses, she adds fresh leaves to wild-peach jam and bitter-orange marmalade. The fresh leaves are preferred whenever there is a choice.

The unobtrusive yellow flowers of bay laurel have no culinary importance, but the small black berries have been used in cooking for two thousand years or more. The taste is said to be similar to that of the leaves. (The name *bay* comes from a Middle English word for "berry," taken from French.)

By its nature, bay is essentially a support to other seasonings, notably in a bouquet of herbs to flavor stocks, braises, and sauces. Despite this near-universal potential, you wouldn't want to meet a bay leaf constantly and everywhere. Unusually, bay stands almost on its own with potatoes, with the help of garlic. (For instance, add six or eight whole cloves of garlic and as many bay leaves to a pan of potatoes to be cooked by browning them in fat in the oven.) In moderation, bay seasons a white sauce (béchamel), depending on the sauce's intended use; the common alternative is nutmeg. Another particular use is in the brine for pickling cuts of pork or corned beef. The flavor of powdered bay is short-lived, but the form is useful for blending into mixtures for meatloaf, meatballs, terrines, pâtés.

The European bay leaves sold today in the United States come not from Europe but from near the Mediterranean coast of Asiatic Turkey. The leaves are gathered in mid- to late summer by mountain peasants — picked by hand in the morning and dried in the shade lest they turn brown. The bay grown on Turkey's Black Sea coast is poorer in quality and sold to Eastern Europe. European bay leaves aren't imported from France or Italy, nor for that matter are they grown commercially in California, because of the high labor costs in more industrialized countries. In Turkey, the seasonal work fits the cycle of peasant life.

Turkish leaves have rounder tips than the narrow leaves on my plants and those pictured in gardening books. Possibly, they are a different strain. The taste is close to other European bay leaves I've tried, but examples grown in different parts of the world apparently show some variation in flavor. Dried *Laurus nobilis* leaves grown in a California backyard and given to me by a friend are quite nutmeggy, with a modest amount of oil-and-resin taste, and they are only a very little bitter. Imported Turkish bay leaves are more resiny, with a clear minor note of bitterness that becomes emphatic when the leaf is held in the mouth.

Herbs and spices turn impotent with age, so it is important to buy them from a store with high turnover. If possible, and especially if you are buying ground or powdered items, choose a shop that specializes in herbs and spices and understands quality. At home, store herbs and spices out of the light in closed containers in, if possible, a cool place.

You can, of course, grow your own bay laurel, either in the ground or in a pot, depending on your climate. Where winter temperatures fall below about 10 degrees Fahrenheit, bay must be cultivated in pots or tubs and carried indoors for the winter. The plant is easy to grow, preferring limey, rich but well-drained soil and full sun. Indoors, place it in a sunny window; fertilize moderately in spring and not at all during winter dormancy (when it prefers a cool room and less sun). Let the surface of the soil dry out visibly before watering; bay will stand quite a bit of dryness. Cut the growing tips back to make the plant bushy. Under near-natural conditions, bay puts out its yearly growth in spring and can be trimmed to keep it to pot size. Having little moisture to begin with, bay leaves dry rapidly after they are picked. For gastronomic purposes, less moisture and poorer soil may better replicate Mediterranean conditions and produce more flavorful leaves.

10

The Sweet Orange Carrot

Here hasn't always been an orange carrot, nor has the carrot always been so very sweet. In large parts of Asia purple carrots are common — purple was the color of the first carrot. If the theory is true that a cultivated plant originated in the place that still has the greatest diversity of types, then the carrot came from Afghanistan. We know about Afghan carrots because Russian scientists investigated wild and domestic carrots there in the 1920s. Besides purple carrots, colored by anthocyanins, the Russians found Afghan carrots that were yellow from anthochlor and mildly orange from carotene.

Much of the arcane history of carrots was written in the 1950s and 1960s by Otto Banga, Dutch carrot specialist. The carrot, the purple carrot, was perhaps first cultivated around the sixth century. During the ninth and tenth centuries, possibly earlier, the carrot spread through the Islamic world. In the classical period, Greek and Roman writers refer to a cultivated carrot of some kind, but they don't mention color and don't seem to have thought much of it as food; this type seems to have died out. A tenth-century account tells of a yellow as well as a purple carrot grown in Babylonia and in Palestine, and the purple is said to have tasted better.

Probably from Islamic Spain or Sicily, carrots entered Italy and then northern Europe. Clues are sparse, but by the fourteenth century carrots were commonly grown outside towns in Holland. By the fifteenth century they were in England. At an uncertain point, perhaps in the Arab world, a white carrot was developed, probably from the faintest yellow. The fourteenth-century *Ménagier de Paris* describes carrots as red roots sold in markets in bunches, one white root per bunch. ("*Carroictes sont racines rouges que l'en vent es Halles par pongnees, et chascune pongnee ung blanc.*") Unfortunately, there is no way to know whether this was a white carrot or a parsnip, since historically carrots and parsnips were sometimes considered as one. But from other sources it seems clear that "red" here signifies purple, in the same way we call beets or red cabbage "red."

In the 1600s, thanks to Dutch painters, carrot history becomes less opaque. The extraordinary century of Rembrandt and Vermeer (and Hals, ter Borch, Cuyp, Hobbema, de Hooch, van Ruisdael) was a time of prosperity in Holland, and artists turned from formalized portraits of the aristocracy to everyday subjects, to appeal to the merchants who were now their customers. Otto Banga found a few paintings by lesser artists that helpfully depict carrots, so we can see how over a period of decades they changed from pale to increasingly bright orange. Dutch prosperity not only supported market gardens but encouraged breeding by vegetable growers, who repeatedly selected the most orange of individual carrots and, we can assume, the best-tasting.

It may be that orange won out because orange food is simply more visually appealing than purple. The orange of carrots also doesn't bleed in cooking, as the red of beets does. Bleeding leaves the purple carrot root unattractively dingy, since it contains less purple anthocyanin than a beet, which does retain a handsome rich color after cooking. Carotene's orange is the most durable of vegetable pigments, especially compared to chlorophyll's green, which turns olive drab in a covered pot or after cooking too long. Anthocyanins produce most reds and purples in plants, and carotene or its relatives produce most yellows and oranges, but also the reds in tomatoes and bell peppers — hence they retain vivid colors even after long cooking.

The carrot that was improved in Holland spread slowly to other countries. European herbalists refer to "red" carrots from the 1500s to the 1700s, but those are still red in the sense that beets are. The herbalists also speak of yellow carrots. The French were probably the most enthusiastic carrot eaters, and like the Dutch they became important breeders. Confusingly, today Europeans still describe orange carrots as "red," and the American variety Red-cored Chantenay is, of course, orange. As late as 1699 John Evelyn, the English diarist, wrote of carrots in *Acetaria*, his noted book on salads, that "the best are yellow."

Americans were late in embracing the carrot. We don't seem to have received the latest improvements. In the eighteenth century, *A Treatise on Gardening, by a Citizen of Virginia* refers to carrots of "two sorts, the orange and the white . . . the former generally used though the latter is much the sweetest." We were likely to consider carrots to be animal feed, matured to a huge size like our eighteenth-century-and-later beets, turnips, or radishes — even those used for human food. Only after the First World War did American enthusiasm for carrots develop. From 1923 to 1953, production increased tenfold.

Joseph Harris, founder of Harris Seeds, wrote a number of farm and garden manuals (including *Walks and Talks on the Farm, Harris on the Pig, Talks on Manure*). His *Gardening for Young and Old*, 1882, contains this aside on the carrot:

> The carrot is not a popular crop. Horses are very fond of carrots, but then they never had to weed them. If they had been obliged to get on their hands and knees, so to speak, with the hot sun on their backs, and had to weed and thin carrots, when Tom and Dick were gone a fishing, they would have been satisfied with dry corn and hay. Boys ought to know better [than horses]. If we want a good thing we have got to work for it. . . . [A] good horse that behaves himself, and cheerfully does all that we ask of him, is entitled to an occasional feed of fresh juicy carrots to mix with his dry hay and corn. But I am sure our bright American boys will soon learn to make the horse do

nine-tenths of the work of raising the carrots. Just think of it! When I was a boy, we used to make a bed about five feet wide, trim it off at the edges with a sharp spade, throw the soil on top from the alleys, rake the bed, and then sow the carrot seed broadcast, and make the bed smooth by patting it with the back of the spade. These beds of carrots, onions, etc., looked very neat and trim when first made, but oh! the labor of weeding them!

(Harris wanted horse-drawn equipment to accomplish nearly every outdoor task.)

The carrot root grows from the point where the often-yellowish core meets the deeper orange outer layer, called the cortex. Because growth occurs at this ring (actually a cylinder within the cylinder of the carrot), the oldest parts of the carrot are just beneath the outer skin and at the very center of the core. Within the core are pathways that carry the sap (nutrients and water) to the leaves; other pathways in the surrounding cortex (for lack of an everyday word) carry the sugars produced in the leaves down to be stored in the root. These up and down vessels are the same (xylem up, phloem down) as those beneath the bark and in the sapwood of a tree; in the cross section of a beet they are arranged as concentric rings (dark xylem and narrower, lighter bands of phloem).

The core of inferior carrots is less sweet and flavorful than the cortex, but plant breeders have worked to erase the taste difference between the two and produce a carrot that is deep orange, crisp, tender, and sweet throughout. In the best carrots they have nearly succeeded.

The carrot belongs to the parsley family (sometimes called the carrot family), which is botanically part of the Umbelliferae (sometimes called the Apiaceae). The flowers are typically umbels: florets on miniature stalks that recall the umbel's etymological kin, the umbrella. Queen Anne's lace, the wild white umbellifer with the central spot of red-black, found through much of North America, is no more than the cultivated carrot, escaped and reverted to primitive form. There is an escaped wild carrot nearly everywhere in the world that carrots are grown. Both kinds are *Daucus carota* and are biennial. The cooked wild root is less sweet and somewhat bitter, with a woody core — bleak compared with the domesticated carrot.

Besides the flower and the typically hollow stem, the general type of an umbellifer is suggested by the form of other culinary members of the family, with their finely cut leaves and aromatic roots, foliage, and seeds. Those include angelica, anise, caraway, celery, chervil, coriander (cilantro), dill, fennel, lovage, parsley, parsnips, samphire (the tender leaves are eaten, often pickled), sea holly (tender shoots and the roots are eaten), and skirret (an old, out-of-favor root).

Carrot flavor often divides into two sorts: a delicate, fresh one from juicy young carrots picked early in the season, and a concentrated one from mature carrots. Young carrots quickly develop carroty flavor while their sugar is still accumulating and their color is pale. Unlike fruit, carrots have no fleeting moment of ripeness. Carrot varieties tend to be best for one or the other kind of flavor. The fresh young carrot that tastes delicious raw is often merely mild when cooked; a more mature carrot does better cooked, though a really old one can be unpleasant.

As with the flavor of tomatoes and nearly every edible plant, the dominant influence on the flavor of a carrot is its variety, its genetic makeup. Phil Simon, a USDA carrot breeder who works at the University of Wisconsin, says that most of the flavor is either sweetness or "harshness," a quality sometimes identified as turpentiney. (Someone I know who eats carrots every day for lunch calls this geranium.) A little provides some essential carrot taste; too much, especially without the soothing effect of sweetness, is repellent. The "harsh" compounds are turpenoids, and some of the same ones occur in pine needles. Phil Simon doesn't consider the compounds to be actually bitter. (True bitterness develops when carrots are stored with a crop, such as apples, that releases ethylene gas as part of ripening.)

Harshness is not exactly a flavor, but a way of summing up the effect of too many turpenoids: both flavor and literal harshness, or irritation. In low levels this may be hard to distinguish from bitterness. We perceive irritation and other mechanical aspects of taste through what is called the trigeminal sense. Texture, such as the crunch of a carrot, is a part of it. An old carrot can be so fibrous as to be woody; a dry one turns rubbery. A crisp, tender raw carrot is ideal.

You might think that there is a relationship between intense orange color and a sweet good taste, but the genetic link between color and flavor is weak, not a consideration at all for plant breeders. A wan carrot may well have been a victim of cold temperatures or some other misfortune while growing. However, strong orange color is directly connected to nutrition, since the body turns carotene into vitamin A. The more orange, the more vitamin A. It is relatively easy for a breeder to increase carotene and thus create a more healthful, deeper orange carrot.

Whatever a carrot's aesthetic qualities, for commercial growers the vegetable must be physically rugged. "Growers handle 'em like they're hammer handles," says Simon. Some of the crisp types found in home gardens are impossible to grow commercially. One breeder puts it that the practical standard may as well be that a carrot should stand being dropped five feet onto a concrete floor, because that's what often happens.

Phil Simon tests the flavors of different carrots against the reactions of tasting panels. Some European tasters have found certain US-developed carrots too sweet, but no American tasters have balked at sweetness. The sugars are primarily glucose and fructose. Everyone has met the taste of glucose and fructose in the quite different context of honey.

The amount of sugar in carrots can be problematic in cooking. In a carrot soufflé, the danger is too much carroty sweetness, which is made worse by onions, sweet enough in themselves. As many cooks know, the taste of sugar is exaggerated by heat and diminished by cold. A frozen dessert requires more sugar than a hot one; a sweet wine is chilled to bring it into balance.

The novice taster quickly latches onto sweetness, which is the taste most people are likely to approve, the only one we have an inborn liking for, except possibly salt. The urge for sweetness probably derives from good biological reasons, since what the body really craves — needs — is calories, not flavor, according to those who study the chemical senses of smell and taste. Conversely, we have an innate dislike of bitterness, but beyond these we learn our likes and dislikes and superimpose them on raw appetite. Our desire for particular flavors is the result of the intervention of mind. But I'm not sure that anyone knows to what extent a taster searches out added sweetness in a carrot and to what extent he prefers a carrot to taste like a carrot — like the learned flavor he already knows.

Only the four basic tastes — sweet, sour, bitter, and salty — are perceived in the mouth, though some would argue for the addition of other tastes, such as metallic or the meaty taste known in Japanese as *umami* and represented by MSG. The rest of flavor is aroma, perceived by smelling before tasting or through vapors rising from the back of the mouth into the nose. The complex interaction between the two senses is little understood, but certainly the mind creates the impression of an array of flavors in the mouth.

It is no coincidence that a number of the scientists who study flavor are psychologists. Linda Bartoshuk is a psychologist at Yale who studies the perception of sweetness. The first thing I learned when I spoke to her is that the well-known map of the tongue, showing exactly where we are supposed to be sensitive to sweet, sour, bitter, and salty, is plain wrong — however often it has appeared in print. She traces the map to an old error. In 1901 a German named Hänig, student of Wilhelm Wundt, father of experimental psychology, wrote a thesis for which he measured sensitivity to the four tastes by dabbing samples of them in spots around the tongue. Hänig drew a graph revealing that the differences among the various locations were actually slight. But a Harvard scientist misunderstood the graph and reported the differences as large, and the mistaken data were seen by someone else to suggest a map of the tongue. The map was made and the mistake perpetuated because for years no one repeated the experiment. The truth is that all our taste buds respond well to all tastes.

The taste buds are arranged in an oval around the tongue, Linda Bartoshuk explains, leaving the center bare. The bumps covering the tongue are called papillae, and the taste buds are buried within certain of them. Three kinds of papillae make up the oval: parallel lines along the sides, large bumps at the back of the tongue, and quite small ones in front. (The papillae in the center without taste buds are a fourth kind.)

Linda Bartoshuk calls the gourmet's taste for particular foods "eccentric" in that it has nothing to do with physiological needs. The gourmet's preferences are strongly influenced by other epicurean opinion, but, she says, these acquired sensitivities, the skills used in making distinctions, are real, along with the pleasure taken. She makes the comparison to an appreciation for music, "subtlety for its own sake."

To return to the carrot, I would say that if the gourmet has perhaps learned to have less taste for sugar than most Americans, a portion of sugar is part of the definition of a carrot. Somewhere between harshness and sweetness each of us finds an area of delicious balance.

As a rule, the higher the sugar content, the more people will like a particular food, but individual sensitivity to sweetness and bitterness varies genetically. People who are moderately sensitive to sweetness find there is no point at which sweetness becomes too cloying and intense; those who are very sensitive often encounter sweet foods that are achingly sweet. As with salt, cooks must know their own inclinations and try to season for the average palate.

Carrots grown in Florida were found by Phil Simon's tasting panels to be almost without sweetness. Florida nights aren't cool enough to slow respiration (oxidation), and sugar is dissipated instead of stored. My father, who lives near Washington, D.C., says that the carrots for sale there are poor compared with the ones in stores around me in Vermont; his are very likely Florida carrots. California, Texas, and Michigan are other states that are major producers. In summer, Quebec has a big share of the fresh market in the Northeast, including Vermont. And the supermarket carrots around here are fairly good.

Rarely is any specific carrot flavor other than sweetness advertised in garden catalogs. The extreme in sugary variety names must be "Orange Sherbet" and "Candy Pak," mentioned in a recent catalog from Stokes Seeds in Buffalo. The same catalog goes so far as to claim there is a "Super Sweet gene," like the two different kinds that were found a few years ago and introduced into new types of sweet corn. For carrots, such genes just don't exist. Unlike the sugar in corn, the sugar in carrots doesn't turn to starch after picking.

If the carrot variety is a tasty one, and if the carrot is freshly picked or carefully stored and not too old when it was picked, its growing conditions determine just how good it is. The best roots are grown at between 60 and 70 degrees Fahrenheit. Above or below, the flavor, texture, and orange color are less good. Higher temperatures produce shorter roots; lower ones encourage longer ones. And too little moisture slows growth, tending to produce more fibrous, resinous, and less sweet roots. A high sodium and calcium soil content, as is found in soil reclaimed from the sea in the Netherlands and in some alkaline California soils, may increase sweetness. Interestingly, quality isn't harmed when carrots grow close together, say an inch apart. Then the roots gain flavor and color faster and at a smaller size, with less of the cracking that sometimes occurs.

Ideal storage conditions are 32 degrees Fahrenheit and 95 percent or more humidity. Because of the sugars, the roots don't freeze until the temperature falls several more degrees. At markets, the foliage of very fresh carrots with their tops still on should be vital, never limp. Mass-marketed carrots with tops removed are often superior to bunched carrots with their tops on; evaporation through the leaves dehydrates and depletes the roots.

So far there is no financial incentive for one grower to produce a higher-quality carrot than anyone else's. No standard for quality exists besides the grower's own. Brands of vegetables, which would enable a grower's superior product to be identified and remembered by the consumer, are just beginning to appear. But brands would make it difficult for a small grower to market his crop independently.

In the 1820s in *The Virginia House-wife*, Mary Randolph prescribed the method for boiling carrots: "Let them be well washed and brushed, but not scraped; an hour is enough for young spring carrots; grown carrots must be cut in half, and will take from an hour and a half to two hours and a half. When done, rub off the peels with a clean coarse cloth, and slice them in two or four, according to their size. The best way to try if they are done enough is to pierce them with a fork." Older recipes, especially French ones, call for halving mature carrots and prying out their woody, poorly flavored cores, either before or after cooking. They may call for parboiling old carrots before going on to the regular cooking, or they may specify impressively long cooking times. Fortunately, with today's carrots we can ignore this advice. The core is often so finely textured and indistinct as to be impossible to separate anyway.

Except for young carrots with mild skin, carrots should be peeled, possibly after cooking, as Mrs. Randolph said. Age and storage produce strong-tasting bitter skin. Actually the taste is mostly aroma, as you can tell very easily by eating carrot skin while pinching your nose. The green shoulders, sometimes reddish purple, that often appear on carrots are also strong and acrid. In the garden this greenness can be prevented by keeping the shoulders covered with soil.

In the days when carrot varieties were less sweet than they are now, sugar was commonly added to the cooking water. I find carrots with added sugar repulsive. Sometimes now the problem is the opposite one. To distract from natural sweetness, the usual additions are salt, lemon juice, vinegar, or the flavor of browning. Or the carrots are diluted by combining them with potatoes. And they can be garnished with crème fraîche, sliced onion, finely chopped fresh chives, hot capsicum pepper. Carrots become even more sweet when all their juices are cooked away.

The flavors for which carrots show the strongest affinity are those of chervil, parsley, tarragon (there is some danger of pointing up a licorice sweetness with that), thyme, and dill; chives and garlic and any member of the onion family; nuts, particularly walnuts; mushrooms; lemon; red-wine vinegar; mustard; salty foods such as ham, olives, pickles, sardines, anchovies, and piquant cheeses (cheddar, provolone, Parmesan, Romano, etc.); and well-browned meats and meat juices. Carrots' balancing effect on other flavors and their liquid mildness find them a place on a platter of antipasti. And like other sweet things, carrots go with spice, as in carrot cake or curried carrots. Perhaps most important, carrots are part of the aromatic underpinning — *mirepoix, soffritto,* etc. — of stocks, many sauces, braises, and a variety of other dishes.

The greatest divide in carrot flavor is between raw and the concentrated taste produced by browning in fat for serving with roasted and grilled meats. The easiest way to cook the vegetable is to "sweat" the sliced roots: to stew them slowly in their own juices with a small amount of oil or butter (about two teaspoons to a pound) in a heavy pot with a tight lid. Carrots can be cooked in advance and held; reheating does little harm. They can be sautéed, boiled, puréed, gratinéed, made into soufflé, cooked in cream, glazed in butter and their cooking juices or added stock, grated and dressed with lemon juice, set with egg and molded in a loaf, boiled and marinated as salad. There isn't much that hasn't been done to a carrot.

Carrot seed, like the seed of anise, caraway, fennel, and other umbellifers, is aromatic, though it has rarely been used as a flavoring. Crushed, it smells of pine, black pepper, and spice generally as well as releasing the vegetable aroma of carrot. Carrot tops are an old esculent, and though they may deserve to be forgotten, it is worth sampling a tender inner frond.

Two particular varieties of carrot emerged in Holland in the 1600s, the Long Orange and the Horn (perhaps named for the city of Hoorn), which are the source of almost all our finest eating carrots today. From Horn came the Nantes carrot, developed over 125 years ago in the French city of Nantes. In the 1940s, eight varieties were important in the United States: Long Orange, Scarlet Horn, Danvers, Oxheart, Red-cored Chantenay, French Forcing, Nantes, and Imperator (a cross between Nantes and Chantenay released in 1928), but only the descendants of Nantes and Imperator are significant commercial varieties today. There was a big advance in sweetness and quality in the United States in the 1960s, much of it the work of Clint Peterson of the USDA.

The "baby" carrots called French Forcing were bred for growing in hothouses, such as those outside Paris, where much breeding was done in the nineteenth century. The beds were heated by the rapid decay of fresh manure (plentifully supplied by horses in those days) beneath six inches of soil. Roots had to be shallow to avoid the hot manure, and any produce given such expensive treatment had to grow quickly and command a high price. The final expression of the breeders' work was the one-and-a-half-inch spherical carrot, now often called Paris Market. An old USDA publication says that it was introduced here in 1861 and that a Round Yellow and a Round White had been developed in France a century earlier.

Americans prefer long, slim carrots, while Europeans prefer shorter, fatter ones. This may be because they regard a fat carrot as further removed from the thin, irregular, uncouth wild carrot. (I add, perhaps irrelevantly, that now in Japan orange carrots have been bred that are as long as three feet.) Any of the long types require a deep, light-textured soil that is free of stones, common enough in the areas of the United States where carrots are grown on a large scale. But in parts of the world where the soil is hard, shallow, or stony, long carrots will not assume their proper shape, and a short stubby shape grows well.

Most of the best of today's carrots are modified versions of Nantes. One carrot breeder I've spoken to at a wholesale seed house in Idaho takes his carrots home from the company's blocks of "inbred" parents used to produce hybrids. He points out that some of the tastiest varieties are experimental, sometimes numbered but unnamed. Ironically, they may never become supermarket varieties because of the very tenderness that recommends them. Not only do the roots of these truer Nantes types tend to shatter, but the tops are too weak for mechanical harvesting. Many store-bought carrots are good, but the freshest, tastiest young carrots are still those grown from varieties found only in small-scale market gardens or home gardens.

11

On English
and French Mustards

The more powerful prepared mustards mount rapidly to the nose, set the eyes to tearing, and make the forehead prickle. Mustard stimulates the appetite (it is said to increase salivation by as much as eight times) and the skin (as in old-fashioned mustard plasters), and perhaps has an effect on thinking (Dioscorides wrote two thousand years ago that mustard is "virtuous in ridding one of the superfluous moods of the brain"). And it enhances other flavors almost without discrimination. But to investigate it is to court confusion. One of the few books devoted solely to it claims that none of the famous black mustard has been cultivated in England since the Second World War and that one of the three mustard species is the same as pak choi, the edible Chinese rape. Wrong on both counts. Many sources confuse the three mustard species, and nearly all, including the *Larousse gastronomique*, misunderstand mustard's two forms of piquant strength. And they cannot agree on which mustard species is strongest.

Oddly, mustard the plant takes its name from mustard the condiment. The word *mustard* derives from *must*, newly pressed unfermented wine, made fiery — *ardent*, so to speak — with ground mustard seed. The word came to English from French almost seven hundred years ago, presumably along with the condiment, although the Romans may have introduced mustard centuries earlier. Both mustard and black pepper are hot, but where pepper grows only in the tropics, mustard is easily grown in any temperate climate. All that is exotic and redolent of wealth and daring exploration in the history of black pepper is commonplace with mustard.

Mustard is a crucifer, a member of the Cruciferae family that includes turnips, radishes, horseradish, garden cress, and watercress — all of them with a suggestion, or much more, of heat. Nearly all the mustard seed on the world market is grown on the Canadian plains, most of it in the province of Saskatchewan and some in adjacent Alberta and Manitoba. In the United States, a very little is grown in Montana and North Dakota, mostly under contract to Canadians. The dry climate of the northern plains ensures good weather during the harvest, and methods of production are similar to those for the grain crops grown there. Mustard, too, is harvested with a combine. In Europe, the price of land demands that farmers grow a more lucrative crop or achieve a very high yield. English mustard yield is three times Canadian. These days, the only European country apart from Britain with a significant crop of mustard is Hungary.

The three mustard species used for the condiment are, or were, known most often by their European names: white (*Sinapis alba*), black (*Brassica nigra*), and brown (*Brassica juncea*). The husk covering the seed of the white is actually a pale tan-yellow; the husk of the black is a dark purplish red-brown; and the husk of the brown varies from brown to as dark as the black, yet it can also be yellow. I obtained samples of the three kinds of mustard in North American commerce, which are called yellow, brown, and oriental (the "oriental" is more yellow than the "yellow"). But the colors were confusing. Did I have examples of the three species? Which seed belonged to which species? Beneath their husks all mustard seeds are yellow, and with husks removed all produce a yellow paste. I spoke with mustard brokers at two Canadian companies that contract with farmers to grow seed and that sell seed to the corporations that produce major American and European brands. Both brokers had their nomenclature straight on the yellow: it is the same as the white (*alba*). But, as I later discovered, they were badly mistaken about the others. Unfortunately, at first I put their information together with some French and English writings and concluded that the black (*nigra*) was characteristic of Dijon and Bordeaux mustards, although mixed with brown (*juncea*). I also accepted at face value the opinion expressed in several books that the black was the most highly regarded and "aromatic."

But I wasn't wholly convinced, and I reached a mustard breeder at the University of Saskatchewan in Saskatoon who avowed that no farmer grew black mustard. Black mustard was a "weed plant" with "no shattering resistance at all," so the seed would scatter when anyone attempted to harvest it. It had "all the characteristics of wild mustard." What the brokers had called black is actually *juncea*. North Americans grow only white and *juncea*. And confusingly, the species *juncea* (which used to be called brown) comes in either a dark-husked type, now called brown in North America, or a yellow-husked type, now called oriental. This breeder also rejected some of the scientific synonyms for the white as plain wrong. His colleague agreed with him about the confusion over names: "Really, you know, it's a mess." Roughly as much white mustard (*alba*) is grown as *juncea*, and the location where the mustard is grown and the season's weather are more important influences on quality than the particular variety.

Having failed to penetrate to a knowledgeable expert at an American company, I turned to Colman's in Norwich, England, largest mustard producer in the world and a user of Canadian mustard as well as English. Colman's promptly connected me with John Hemingway, who had retired from Colman's not long before and become a private international consultant. He is the world's greatest mustard expert.

The English mustard tradition is represented by Colman's clean, sharp, strong yellow powder — historically, a blend of black and white. Black mustard originated in Asia Minor and Iran, and, as I quickly learned, for more than twenty-five years it has scarcely been grown because of that inability to submit to a mechanized harvest. A tiny amount comes on the market from Ethiopia, Sicily, India, and

Nepal. But all of Colman's dark mustard seed was black, grown in England, until 1954, when the first crop of *juncea* was planted. Then *juncea* rapidly replaced black both in England and on the Continent, where some proportion of black had been used in Dijon, Bordeaux, and other mustards. (Black mustard seed is smaller than the familiar white, which is used in pickles and relishes.) John Hemingway says, "*Nigra* never was as good as all that." Any dark seed called black nowadays is all but certainly *juncea*. And black "does nothing that *juncea* can't do far better." What is the source of the lingering belief in its superiority? Perhaps, "Absence makes the heart grow fonder."

On the species of mustard and their types, John Hemingway agrees, "People do get into an awful muddle." *Juncea* originated in the Himalayan area and was disseminated from three secondary areas: one in China; one in the Crimea; and one encompassing India, Pakistan, and Bangladesh (this *juncea* has a cabbagey flavor and makes distasteful mustard, although the seed is an important source of cooking oil in these countries). The first two are the sources of the *juncea* now grown in Europe and North America and distinguished by Americans as brown or oriental. *Juncea* is the mustard found in Chinese restaurants, and certain varieties are grown for salad greens. John Hemingway, who admires precision, doesn't approve of the name *oriental*, since the origins of the type are not necessarily oriental. Many varieties were developed by Colman in England. Awkwardly, the only clear way now to refer to the species as a whole is by its scientific name.

White mustard is an eastern Mediterranean native, and like the other kinds it is widely naturalized in North America. It is planted as a green-manure crop for tilling into the ground to improve the soil. (The yellow flowers of white, black, or *juncea* mustards are a familiar sight in fields, where they are sometimes regarded as a nuisance.) White mustard is the kind used in American ballpark mustard, of which the original is French's, dyed bright yellow, flavored by turmeric, and above all mild. It succeeded exactly because in 1904 Francis French deduced that Americans weren't buying much mustard because they didn't like it hot. But, of course, to many people heat is the main point of mustard.

The English attachment to mustard is old and passionate. Very long ago, mustard seed was put on the table like salt; the eater crushed the seed on the bare board with the handle of his knife and sprinkled it over his food. But at an early date the prepared condiment was common as well. Wrote Florence White in *Good Things in England*, "Every day in the 16th century and earlier, brawn with mustard was the first dish served at the twelve o'clock dinner from November to February." This mustard was coarsely ground like some of today's. Continues Miss White, "The black mustard, which is the best, grows wild in England and was most likely used as a condiment by the Saxons. It was cultivated in gardens in the 16th century in the neighborhood of Tewkesbury, ground up and made into balls and sent to London." Portions were broken off and, relying still on Miss White, mixed with "wine vinegar" or "grape or apple juice, ale, buttermilk, white wine, claret, or the juice of cherries" — to make mustard for the table. (Falstaff says in *Henry IV*, "His wit is as thick as Tewkesbury mustard.") But Tewkesbury mustard has since disappeared without a trace.

The popularizer of smooth English mustard from fine powder was Mrs. Clements of Durham. About 1720, she was inspired to mill mustard seed, likely with a wooden stamper, and strain it through a series of progressively finer bolting cloths, exactly as if she were a miller producing white flour from wheat. She was not the first to have the idea (in 1600 Sir Hugh Plat recommended more or less the same procedure in *Delightes for Ladies*). But Mrs. Clements acted on it and, according to lore, managed to keep her method secret, so that she built up a highly profitable mustard business. She sold her Durham mustard to George I. It is reasonable to assume that she blended black and white mustard flours, since that was already a long-established habit.

Jeremiah Colman, who gave his name to the famous English mustard business, was the successful owner of a windmill by the Magdalen Gate in Norwich, where he produced animal feeds. In 1814, he rented a second, water-powered, mill four miles away in Stoke Holy Cross. This happened to be both a grist- and a mustard mill, and thus Jeremiah Colman entered the mustard business. The mustard was ground in water-powered stampers, now in the Mustard Museum in Norwich. Mr. Colman, like Mrs. Clements, mastered the skill of grinding mustard fine without heating it and bringing out the oil. (Black mustard is in the range of 30 percent oil.) The company thrived and expanded, and in 1866, Colman's was appointed mustard-maker to Queen Victoria. John Hemingway says, "Personally, I think that what Mr. Colman succeeded in doing was to make mustard the natural third condiment — salt, pepper, and mustard." This occurred in the Victorian and Edwardian eras. "In my grandfather's time, it was always open salt, pepper pot, mustard pot, in a silver stand." By 1926, Colman's was in a position to buy the R.T. French Company in the United States, where Colman's sales had been weak.

Colman's English mustard is today a blend of roughly equal parts of white and *juncea* (formerly black) mustard flours, ground separately by steel rollers and sifted free of husks through silk bolting cloths. Most of the seed is grown by contract with English farmers in the drier eastern counties of the country. Colman's produced and sold only powder until 1933, when it offered prepared English mustard, the first foodstuff ever put into a tube. Besides fresh potency, the advantage to home-mixed Colman's powder over a ready-mixed mustard is that the powder can be added to food without adding sugar, vinegar, and other flavorings at the same time.

Flavor, as it is usually defined, is a combination of the tastes in the mouth (sweet, sour, bitter, salty) with the aromas sensed in the nose. By this definition, flavor is distinct from mustardy heat and pungency, which are perhaps better understood as irritation, or a kind of mechanical reaction. Mustard seeds aren't usually credited with flavor. The way to see for yourself is to chew the seeds while holding your nose, until the heat or pungency asserts itself, then release your nose to see if the flavor expands. I find a slight flavor of grain. The interaction among taste, aroma, and perhaps heat and pungency produces a much greater effect than do the separate parts.

Chewing plain whole mustard seeds, you taste at first little more than a faint sweetness, then a small amount of heat appears and develops. No mustard has either flavor or fire until the cells are broken and water is added. And then it takes a few moments for the potency to show and about twenty minutes to achieve full force. The enzyme myrosin precipitates a chemical reaction that produces one substance (acrinyl isothiocyanate) in white mustard and another (allyl isothiocyanate) in black and *juncea* mustards.

The two chemicals have different effects. White mustard heats only the tongue. Black and *juncea* mustards can be felt on the tongue but they rise memorably to the nose, eyes, and even the forehead. Their pungency is more intense than that of the white and longer lasting once the condiment is mixed. Mixing with hot water limits or prevents the chemical reactions, and mixing with vinegar or another acid inhibits them. *Juncea* almost requires mixing with vinegar to lessen its force. (The hot compound in *juncea* is the same as the one in horseradish and in watercress.) I believe that the reason the mustards served in North American Chinese restaurants are so powerful is that they are freshly mixed with water only. Once the paste is made and heat and pungency are formed, adding acid helps to preserve them in the jar.

The British combination of white with black or *juncea* provides the full teasing effect of both strong mouth heat and nasal awakening. One can only speculate on the cultural reasons for the British preference for the combined power and for strong mustard to boot. Colman's mustard sells well in former parts of the British Empire and in Japan, where the admiration for pungency is old. French styles of mustard sell well in parts of the world inhabited by Latins.

The highly opinionated and usually perceptive English writer

Morton Shand, who lived most of his life as an expatriate in France, dissented from his countrymen's taste. "Our national, water-made mustard is a piteously amateur business, thin as buttermilk.... Flavour, of course, it has none. It burns.... Mustard-powder should be banished from every self-respecting English home, unless it is kept in close proximity to a bottle of good wine-vinegar and access to the tap for its confection has been sternly forbidden the cook." On the other hand, he found French mustard "deliciously mild and suave, but at the same time full of a piquant and stimulating relish that lends a warming, insinuating fillip to the flavour to which it is lent." Morton Shand was unfair, but at least he raised the question of the gastronomic role of mustard's heat and pointed to the achievements of the Burgundian *moutardiers*.

In France, mustard-making is an ancient craft. In 1292, there was a guild of ten mustard-makers in Paris, whose activities were restricted to making and selling the condiment. The history of French mustard has less to do with technology and more with the relationship between mustard and the liquid that makes it a sauce. The French have never made powdered mustard (with one or two failed exceptions). Mustard-makers and vinegar-makers were from the earliest period often one and the same. The preferred seed has always been dark, either black or brown, and it was and is mixed with an acid, usually vinegar. It was soaked in the acid before grinding, drained, and mixed with it again afterward. The old French device was a mustard quern, a pair of stones, the top one turned by hand using a wooden *bâton*, which made a grim daylong task for a worker. The Industrial Revolution altered English mustard-making sooner than the French; hand methods were replaced in France only late in the nineteenth century. In Dijon, after grinding, the husks were filtered out of the wet mustard (they are now centrifuged) to create a smooth yellow paste. If the husks are left in and ground fine, mustard is brown, as are coarse mustards from dark seed. The choice of liquid also affects color; clear liquids show the mustard color, while red-wine vinegar muddies it.

Mustard, like black pepper, offers a fairly noncommittal heat, a background for a number of flavorings, some of the most successful being subtle blends of herb and spice that are nearly impossible to identify individually. An ancient alliance is mustard with another source of heat — horseradish, black pepper, chilies, green peppercorns — which counterposes the different sources of heat and whatever there is of taste and aroma as well. But the effect always seems to be to enhance the mustard. The flavors are generally melded and the heat is tempered by brief aging, traditionally in wood, before the mustard is sold.

Dijon mustard, not all of which is nowadays made in the city of Dijon, is perhaps as old as any. As long ago as 1390 under Philip the Bold, duke of Burgundy, an ordinance was passed to regulate Dijon vinegar-mustard makers. Mustard seed had to be soaked in and mixed with only good vinegar and aged for twelve days before it was sold. At various periods, must was the liquid. During the eighteenth century, Dijon vinegar had apparently declined to a corrupt fluid; a maker named Jean Naigeon was hailed for his innovation of replacing vinegar with verjuice, the juice of very sour unripe grapes. In 1742 white-wine vinegar was first used, and about that time additions of capers and anchovies first appeared. Into the twentieth century, a separate variety of white grape was grown for verjuice, but the most common liquid in Dijon mustard has nearly always been vinegar.

Innumerable firms have made mustard in France. Most of the famous companies of the last hundred years — Bocquet, Bordin, Dessaux Fils, Les Frères Gros, Parizot, Raffort — have collapsed into one another, leaving a few dominant concerns, though they maintain many of the old names. One famous firm is Maille, founded in 1747. At its peak of inventiveness in the nineteenth century, Maille offered twenty-four flavors of mustard and ninety-two of vinegar. That French house is now owned by Grey-Poupon (or vice versa, due to the shifting corporate umbrella), which was itself founded in 1777, although Maurice Grey came years later and Auguste Poupon joined him only in 1866. Grey supplied mustard to the court of Napoleon III, and in 1850 he created automatic machinery to replace the hand operation of the old querns.

The right to manufacture Grey-Poupon in the United States is now owned by Nabisco. The jar label, like others, reveals no secrets; it says "based on the original Dijon, France, recipe." One of the few facts disclosed by the head of corporate communications is that the seeds pass through a French mustard mill. The technical people "don't talk about this product at all," and the recipe is kept locked in a safe. But a careful taster will suspect tarragon and chervil and perhaps clove or allspice. Mustard manufacturers wouldn't have proliferated in the past (158 were active in Paris alone in the year Grey-Poupon was founded) if the procedure and flavorings were truly secret. It is, in fact, simple to soak, grind, and variously flavor the whole seeds yourself at home (don't grind unsoaked seeds in a food processor) to produce a coarse mustard, and various mustard powders can be bought for mixing. Acquiring a famous name has more to do with marketing than manufacture. In the case of Nabisco's Grey-Poupon, there is added cachet from the use of white wine, noted prominently on the jar, although it is indistinguishable from the vinegar and water listed first as ingredients.

Bordeaux mustard (Louit is the famous name) is dark from the husks, sweet, and flavored with spices and herbs. Mustard has also been made in Orleans, Beaune, Reims, and many French cities. The coarse mustard from Meaux, east of Paris, was first made by monks in the 1600s; it became Meaux de Pommery a century later when it was bought by the Pommery family. Brillat-Savarin is supposed to have said, "The only mustard is Meaux." Philip the Good said over three hundred years before, "The only mustard is in Dijon."

The black seed used during most of the period of French mustard manufacture was probably grown in France, though in time seed was also imported from other countries. By the late nineteenth century, increasing amounts of *juncea* were used, and at least some white mustard came into play. In 1937, a law was passed in France forbidding the use of white mustard except in Alsace and Lorraine, where white mustard was traditional. (Actually, white is permissible everywhere, but the paste may be labeled only *"condiment."*) The French have sometimes accused white mustard of being bitter and creating a persistent heat in the mouth. But the primary explanation offered for banning the white was that it lacked the pungent chemical that affects the nose. Ironically, these days French makers produce milder mustards for export than they do for consumption at home.

In England, William Tullberg is a mustard-maker who has revived old, coarse-grained styles. In 1970 he began making mustard and then founded Wiltshire Tracklements, now located in the village of Sherston. As part of his work as a meat wholesaler, he tasted a great many sausages and grew tired of the available mustards. He began to make his own, put up a dozen pots for sale in the local pub, and that was the start of the business. *Tracklement* is a curious word that means "a flavorful adjunct to meat": mustard, onions, herbs, various root vegetables, mint sauce with lamb, applesauce with pork. Says the *Oxford English Dictionary*, "Dorothy Hartley claimed to have invented this word. She also claimed that her use of it in this sense was a specific application of an older word, probably dialect, meaning 'appurtenances, impedimenta,' but no evidence of such a word has been found." Dorothy Hartley spoke of tracklements in the 1950s in her admirable writings about practical and mostly obsolete rural lore.

There are now fifteen Wiltshire Tracklements mustards, all more or less English. Says William Tullberg, "I'd say we returned to the medieval tradition in mustard-making and have expanded it to create a very individual style (now much imitated!). Our own techniques are a marriage of [English and French] and include simultaneous grinding of all dry ingredients and maturing in batches, neither of which is in the 'tradition' of England or France. Having visited English and French factories, I'd say that the major brands are substantially removed from any tradition except the hot pursuit of the franc and the pound!" The white seed for his mustards is grown by a local farmer, who is now making the transition to organic; the *juncea* is Canadian, although Tullberg, not surprisingly, is under the impression that it is the abandoned black species.

I've tasted only five of the Wiltshire mustards: the Black, Strong English (in line with Mrs. Clements's and Jeremiah Colman's work), Devizes Beer, Taunton Cyder, and Spiced Honey. Most contain coarsely ground white or *juncea* mustard or a mix. They are expensive (and, unfortunately, hard to find in the United States), but they do teach you about other possible mustard mixtures than the familiar sorts. You may not focus on the whole of the liquid medium immediately, but the flavor of Farmer's Glory ale from Devizes and of Taunton (hard) cider are quite distinct on retasting. All are buttressed by some wine vinegar or cider vinegar. Other mustards in the line are conventionally flavored with tarragon, green peppercorns, garlic and chives, horseradish. The five I've encountered include all the important ones except the Full Strength, which I'm sorry to have missed. And I like all but the Spiced Honey; I don't care for its sweetness. There is a long history of mixing mustard with honey, and others have liked it best, but even so. . . . The taste for sugar with savory food is a complicated subject related to the beverages you drink with food by habit and to the depth and complexity of flavors you are used to.

I have pondered the role mustard might play with dry, salty aged country ham. The effect of the typical salty mustard, including various Dijons, is more nearly an assault than a subtle marriage of tastes. And the salt can't claim the excuse of preserving mustard's heat or pungency. It doesn't. Says Mr. Tullberg, "I agree with your point about salt and ham. My favorites in our range to accompany a York dry-cure ham would be Cider Mustard and Full Strength, neither of which contains salt. Why? Simply because they didn't feel right or taste right in the context of their other flavorings when salted — the advantage of creating one's own tradition!" His unsalted mustards do work.

Not to disparage the Dijon style. Like most mustards, Dijon

goes best with the milder forms of salted meat — corned beef, fresh sausages, hot dogs, most brine-cured hams (mustard is almost required when these are sugar-cured), pâtés, terrines — and with fresh meats, especially pork and beef with their full meat flavors. Nearly any mustard gives new life to leftover meat. And strong English mustard goes well with cheddar cheese. Mustard is essential to a salad dressing of cream and lemon juice. Some sauces contain clearly recognizable mustard, such as *sauce Robert*, mentioned by Rabelais more than four hundred years ago (onions cooked in fat, with white wine, vinegar, mustard), or *sauce rémoulade* (mustard, chopped pickles, capers, herbs, sometimes anchovy, in a mayonnaise). Just a hint of Dijon mustard helps to bind a sauce as it adds complexity and often-useful acidity, without revealing the source. Mustard shows especially well against cream. Heat destroys mustard's bite, so mustard is added at the end of cooking, if the dish allows. The more potent *juncea* mustard lasts longer in the heat.

The husk, or bran, of the white mustard is mucilaginous and provides thickening to versions of the condiment that contain white mustard; in mustard prepared only from *juncea* some liquid may separate and come to the top. There is, however, nothing wrong with a little separation. The mustard just needs mixing back together. Some mustards contain less bran than others, and bran is sometimes used to stretch less expensive mustards. There are other ways to thicken mustard and cut its intensity besides adding bran, although additions such as wheat flour are sometimes construed as adulterants. The prepared condiment itself, whatever seed is in it, helps to emulsify such sauces as vinaigrette and mayonnaise.

Because of its acidity and, typically, its salt, a bought jar of mustard doesn't spoil, but slowly loses its fire and flavor, even in a vacuum-sealed jar. Heat and pungency begin to decline as soon as they reach their peak twenty minutes after mixing. Therefore, it is unfair to judge a brand if the jar has lingered for months on a store shelf, and one should buy a small enough quantity at a time that it will be used up fairly quickly. (I admit I usually buy mustard only a few times a year, but if I want good flavor for something I buy a new jar.) Part of the problem is oxidation, so an opened jar should be kept capped in a cool pantry or the refrigerator. After a while, mostly acidity is left.

I offer a last provocation from Rosamond Man and Robin Weir, authors of *The Compleat Mustard*. After writing the book, they took a retrospective look at the essential nature of mustard in a brief paper prepared for the 1987 Oxford Symposium on Food. (They had commented in the book, "The problem was not, as so many had asked, whether there was enough to write a book about mustard, but to know how, and when, to stop.") They still wrestled with confusion about species and about heat in the mouth versus pungency in the nose versus taste and aroma, but they had experimented at length with flavoring all kinds of food with mustard. The authors admit to few or no bounds: chocolate "is especially heightened." And they believe mustard enhances sweetness generally, especially in fruit — "mangoes, bananas, strawberries, peaches, dessert apples ... cooked or uncooked." That calls to mind the fruit-mustard combination in *mostarda di Cremona* or *mostarda di Venezia*, rare examples of the modern Italian use of any mustard and almost certainly medieval survivals. Man and Weir claim, after considerable tasting, that mustard enhances the flavor of virtually all other foods — whether or not mustard's own flavor has been lost in the heat of cooking. They speculate that mustard may contain something that acts on flavors in a fashion parallel to MSG.

Perhaps a better point of comparison is black pepper. Both pepper and mustard have character that heightens the flavor of other foods. But while pepper works well in subtle amounts and hardly ever in large ones, mustard is better in definite, even bold quantities. It is excellent with meats, but it competes with or hides the flavor of certain foods, not least that of good olive oil in a vinaigrette (as good as a mustardy vinaigrette is with strong greens). Mustard isn't quite ideal with everything.

Roast Beef

Standing ribs of beef are the most celebratory and essential of roasts. To roast, in the true sense of the word, is to cook on a spit before a radiant fire — gas, electric, or charcoal, but preferably wood. Roasting is the most direct way to cook (there is no intermediary of liquid or fat): it brings out the pure flavor of the meat. The essence of roasting, what defines it, is a deeply caramelized, richly flavored outer crust encasing a succulent and, one hopes, tender interior — cooked no further than rare. That juxtaposition of qualities can be achieved only with high heat. For roast beef, salt and pepper are all the seasonings needed. The most flattering accompaniments are usually simple ones, and there is a case to be made for a thick slice of aged prime rib alone on a plate, constituting an entire course in itself. In restaurants where you pay dearly for a tour de force, you don't find basic roast beef. It isn't on the cutting edge of fashion.

Roast beef is only compromised by sauces, herbs, tomatoes, or garlic. To go with it, there should be plenty of food — it can be a long meal. But it should be a simple one; top quality requires no visual frills and calls for straightforward accompaniments. Winter vegetables, roots, have a special affinity for roasts: potatoes, carrots, turnips, parsnips, the bland and unusual salsify, the underappreciated celeriac; some member of the onion family is almost imperative. Small onions and shallots can be baked whole in their skins and peeled before serving. Vegetables cut in large pieces can be "roasted" in the oven in a pan with drippings taken from the beef or with olive oil. They can also be put in a tightly covered pan over low heat and stewed in a little butter or olive oil. Or, a small variation, cook them with water and some butter in a covered sauté pan and finish by lightly glazing them in their own juices. These methods concentrate flavor.

An unadorned roast is itself a well-known accompaniment to a mature red wine. But happily, roast beef and almost any mellow red wine each clarifies the flavor of the other. The use of sauces, herbs, tomatoes, and garlic, besides altering the natural flavor of ribs of beef, undercuts the subtlety and complexity of an exceptional wine. But with an ordinary wine consider "roasting" potatoes together with whole cloves of unpeeled garlic for their quiet, enriching presence, removing the garlic before serving.

With a more ordinary wine, don't shun horseradish (finely grated, mixed with whipped cream or crème fraîche, and seasoned to taste with salt, a touch of sugar, and lemon juice). A different note is struck by a potato gratin, a *gratin dauphinois* made with cream (but no egg, no cheese) and served either with the roast or beforehand as its own course. Mushrooms are excellent cooked plainly in any fashion. Green beans look cheerful against the warm colors on the plate. But generally, place green vegetables in their own course before or after the main one: a soup, timbale, custard, gratin, salad, already made and designed to keep the cook as host out of the kitchen. Neither asparagus nor artichoke hearts, though both are delicious with roast beef, are a gift to wine: they contradict the premise of a simple food set against the intricacies of a good wine.

Vegetables to accompany the roast should be thoroughly cooked, so as to give almost no resistance to the tooth. (In season and in their perfect youth, make an exception for carrots, turnips, and green beans.) Any sentimental accompaniment makes its own rules; however, fruit, beets, and sweet potatoes are too sweet and out of place with roast beef. Whatever the vegetables are, they should be served from their own dishes rather than placed around the roast on its platter — to save the carver from inadvertently tumbling them onto the table.

Roots are equally good in purée, classical French form. They may appear individually or in improvised combinations. Season them with cooked onions or shallots, and, if necessary, thicken with potato to avoid watery puddles. A purée is rapidly made in a food processor (unless a vegetable, such as celeriac, is woody; in that case, put it through a food mill and then through a fine strainer). A purée of winter squash is tasty.

What is unsurpassed with roast beef is Yorkshire pudding; it is hard to make enough to satisfy those who like it. Hot, it will support a large quantity of delicious fat drippings without tasting heavy. Yorkshire pudding was not always served the way it is today, straight from oven to table, puffed and crisp on top and bottom. Harder (higher protein) flour produces a higher rise. Yorkshire pudding used to be baked and then set for a time beneath the still-turning roast to catch more drippings, as it sometimes still is. And rather than the good, light-tasting modern British style, Escoffier and Montagné (who in the *Larousse gastronomique* called it "a sort of heavy crêpe, rather than a proper pudding") would bake the batter in a smaller, deeper vessel than the wide, shallow British one. That more solid and perhaps traditional result would be cut into diamond shapes in the kitchen and arranged around the roast to decorate it. Of course, all Yorkshire puddings when cool turn heavy.

When Dorothy Sayers finally married off her detective, Lord Peter Wimsey (*Busman's Honeymoon*, 1937), she settled him into a large country house that contained an inadequate Victorian kitchen range along with the requisite crime to be solved. The kitchen problem was solved with the least effort. Lord Peter: "We will take it a few periods back and have it Tudor. I propose to install an open fire and a roasting-spit," to be turned, very reasonably, by electricity. Contrary to Lord Peter's impression, roasting before an open fire persisted up to the time of his Victorian range. Isabella Beeton, in her famous mid-nineteenth-century English cookbook, *Mrs. Beeton's Book of Household Management,* suggests no other way to roast beef.

The difficulty with a spit is its need for turning, preferably slowly and continuously. Turning creates a degree of self-basting as emerging fat and juices run over the surface of the meat before falling to the dripping pan below. The meat must be tightly fastened and spitted dead-on through its center of gravity, or with each rotation it will move at first slowly and then suddenly — so that one side will be done while the other is still nearly raw. When spit roasting was common, the task of turning fell variously to children or to the lowest of kitchen workers — who turned but never judged the meat or fire — or the turning was done by clockwork mechanisms, even dogs on a treadmill.

The skills of managing the fire and determining when the meat is perfectly done have never been taken lightly. According to the over-quoted aphorism of Brillat-Savarin, "We can learn to be cooks, but we must be born knowing how to roast." I disagree. It is much easier and requires no innate talent (no tasting) to learn to roast. And nowadays a thermometer confers a good share of expertise on a neophyte.

One can, and I normally do, "roast" in an oven using very high heat. That is a reasonable compromise with convenience, although a passionate article on roasting in Pierre Larousse's great nineteenth-century encyclopedia refers to "meats traitorously stewed in an oven." Certainly the result is not the same. With a fire, there is plenty of draft to carry away steam. To roast is to cook by radiant heat — dry heat. Oven roasting is really high-heat baking. In oven roasting, the appliance's usual convected currents of damp hot air are partly compensated for by the drying effect of extra heat and the unusual amount of radiant heat emanating from the metal walls. But the steam in the enclosed space doesn't allow the incomparable effects of true roasting.

The lines that distinguish one method of cooking from another are sometimes artificial, but they make the concepts clear. Boiling is obviously not gentle poaching, and sautéing is distinct from deep-fat frying. Baking in a sealed, traditionally masonry, oven surrounds a dish with heat. Roasting takes place *in front of* a fire and grilling takes place *over* it. Unlike grilled steak or sausage, roasted meat should have no taste of smoke or only the barest hint of it. Grilling is a fast way of cooking tender meat cut in relatively thin shapes. (Broiling *beneath* the source of heat, as in the open-front salamander of a commercial range or beneath a home oven broiler with the door ajar, is perhaps a form of roasting.)

A further blurring occurs in oven roasting when meat in contact with the bottom of the pan fries in its own fat. The arc of the ribs, cut long enough, prevents that, and so of course does a metal rack. But with a rack, the pan itself shields the bottom of the meat from so much heat that it cooks more slowly than the rest, even apart from the insulating effect of the bones. With a rack, turn the meat at least once.

The heat of fire or oven should permit the exterior of the meat to finish browning at the same time as the interior is cooked to rare. That is where the skill lies: adjusting the heat of the fire, gauging the distance from fire to roast, knowing when the fire may be allowed to die down — all in relation to the size and especially the thickness of the meat. Naturally, all that requires some experience. A few minutes either way affects doneness, though the meat need not be done literally to a turn. Should basting be required, the open fire allows it without the interruption caused by removing a roast from an oven. Repeated basting enhances the brown glaze, but when the meat is well marbled by fat within and retains a layer of fat without, basting is unnecessary. The fat covering deprives the meat of some of its brown exterior. A thick layer of fat only makes sense if you plan to eat it. But some fat is important, because it bastes the meat as it melts and so aids in browning. This fat won't fatten you unless you help yourself to a nice crisp piece.

The meat is seared for the compelling reason of the deliciousness of the deeply browned crust. Roasting is sometimes done with intense heat first followed by a slow finish, and sometimes by slow initial cooking followed by browning at the end. It is, however, easier to judge doneness when the roasting is quick at the start and gradually slowed, as if the fire were dying, because that way the meat's temperature is rising more slowly at the end and there is a longer period when the inside is at the desired rare state.

For the cook lacking experience, a thermometer reveals interior doneness. The old test of pressing on the meat with a finger is more useful in grilling than in roasting beef. (Flaccid theoretically is rare; some resistance is medium; firm is hopelessly well done. With roasting ribs of beef, you can press on the center of the eye, but it doesn't face the fire directly so it tells little.) Another venerable test works well, although it requires practice and I don't know how to specify the uncomfortably hot state that signifies doneness: insert a metal skewer into the middle of the roast; after a minute, withdraw it and check the heat against your lips. The most certain test is to insert a cook's rapid-response thermometer into the center of the roast, and take the meat from the heat when it registers between 120 and 125 degrees Fahrenheit. (A small disadvantage to either a skewer or a thermometer is that some juice is lost through the opening it creates.) At 125 degrees the juices run pink and clear, not bloody. Once the meat is out of the oven, the internal temperature will rise at least another 5 to 10 degrees. Compensate by removing the meat when it is below the desired point. Doneness up to 140 degrees Fahrenheit, medium, appeals to some people; beyond this point meat is called roast beef only out of kindness to the cook.

The heat during cooking, especially when even from steady turning, drives the juices to the center of the meat, so when it is removed from the heat, it must be left to rest on a warm platter for another twenty to thirty minutes while the juices redistribute themselves. If the roast is carved too soon, it will divide tragically into a pool of juices and slices of dry meat.

There is a method that calls for cooking the beef entirely in a slow oven. That truly is baking and it takes much longer; there is less shrinkage and loss of weight, and little chance of overcooking. But the browning is poor and you never come close to the excitement of a real roast. You can tell when you are served beef that was cooked slowly: the interior is one consistent shade of red except for a very narrow border of brown. You might as well poach the meat instead.

After roasting, the intensely flavored juices that accumulate in the dripping or roasting pan can be degreased and spooned over the meat. Or they can be dissolved in water or wine, strained into a small saucepan, reduced over high heat until they concentrate and thicken, and then spooned over the meat. That can heighten flavor to an extraordinary extent, producing a much cleaner effect than an old-fashioned flour-thickened gravy. Or the juices can be the basis for a more elaborate sauce.

Two things can make American beef especially delicious: feeding cattle on grain and aging the meat after slaughter. The grain is generally corn, which is fed to cattle for 120 to 180 days. Then, if the herd is a good one, 80 percent of the animals will be graded USDA prime or USDA choice. Usually they are eighteen to thirty months old. Grain feeding improves the flavor and increases the amount of fat, which is partly saying the same thing. The marbling of fat within the red meat produces a large part of the distinctive beef taste and on the tongue adds to the impression of juiciness. Animals that are fed on grass or forage (including silage) are leaner, and their fat tends to be yellower. A few people who were brought up on grass-fed beef, which gives what is called a "dairy" or "milky" flavor, prefer it. But most people, including the French, who never used to indulge their cattle in grain, think grain-fed beef tastes better.

A beef carcass is graded by examining the exposed eye of the rib between the twelfth and thirteenth ribs. Thirteen ribs are all there are, and that point is chosen because it divides the forequarter from the hindquarter. The grader determines what is prime mostly according to the abundance of marbling and the age of the animal. To a lesser extent he looks for light red, fine-textured, firm meat.

Darker flesh usually comes from older animals. There are, of course, lean cuts of meat within a prime carcass, and certainly leaner cuts and leaner grades than prime can be roasted. (Generally, the leaner cuts are tougher and less tasty and more suited to braising. Lean or otherwise, only the more tender cuts are appropriate for grilling and sautéing.) The leanest benefit from a marinade, from larding (inserting strips of fat into the lean flesh), or from barding (tying a layer of fat to the outside to prevent it from drying during cooking — the fat is removed before the meat is served).

Prime beef truly is superior. Once a summer guest went to the local butcher to buy a steak. When she saw the thick steak the butcher cut for her, she became confused and had the butcher slice it again into two thin steaks, each merely half an inch thick. They could hardly be passed over the grill without becoming gray all the way through. However, seared over a hot fire on one side, with the other unsightly and barely gray side turned down on the plate, the overcooked meat was still delicious because it was prime and somewhat aged — a testament to the resiliency of good meat. Prime beef isn't exactly health food, but when it does appear it is appreciated in almost any guise.

Another factor that bears on flavor is the breed of the animal. Beef from Angus cattle has been given extra appeal through promotion by the American Angus Association. The group apparently sets higher than usual standards for "certified" Angus beef. But the same standards could be applied to another breed, and a few years ago a spokesman for the organization told me that if you tasted top-quality steaks from Angus and another breed, you wouldn't be able to tell which were which. Others say there may be as much variation of quality within a breed as between breeds. Some individuals may just taste beefier. Much of the difference in taste between traditional breeds, generally named for the regions where they arose, probably comes or came from regional differences in what cattle are or were fed. It's safe to say there is no best breed, only different breeds, whose somewhat different characteristics have been too little considered.

Charolais steaks from France are more blond than typical beef. The famous Florentine *bistecca alla fiorentina* comes from the Tuscan Chianina breed. Beef in American supermarkets used to come from such British beef breeds as Hereford, Angus, and Shorthorn. In the United States, they were bred and interbred to produce more and better beef. At the same time, Continental breeds continued to be developed for multiple uses — as draft animals and for milk and beef. Some of those breeds were larger than American beef cattle. And a couple of decades ago Americans started experimenting with breeds like Charolais, Simmental, Limousin, Salers, and Brahmin, most of them from Europe. Now, anything goes. There is still pure-bred stock, but most herds are well mixed. The beef in the super-market comes from any of fifteen breeds or more. And, of course, the cattle industry is breeding and feeding to produce leaner beef.

An older animal yields tougher but more flavorful meat — as does a well-exercised animal or a well-exercised muscle, like the meat on the shank or neck or tail. (Bill Bridges, in *The Great American Chili Book,* quotes a Californian who says old-timers insisted that "a 13-to-15-year-old Longhorn bull" made the best chili. Clearly, any tenderness was achieved through hours of cooking.) Italian beef and veal are characterized by being slaughtered younger than their American counterparts — one reason why there is no *bistecca alla fiorentina* in the United States.

The tenderness of a rib roast varies from end to end. The cut is usually composed of no more than the seven middle ribs cut from the thirteen. As the ribs grow smaller toward the hindquarter, they are less fatty and more tender.

Most of the prime beef sold to specialty butchers and restau-rants has been given some extra aging beyond the one to two weeks that occurs on the way to market. Sometimes restaurants specify three or four weeks of aging. The outer limit before serious decom-position sets in is about six weeks. Beef is aged at 32 to 34 degrees Fahrenheit in 85 to 90 percent humidity. What occurs is a kind of controlled spoilage, somewhat similar to the ripening of cheese.

Compounds present in the meat begin to digest it, tenderizing it and changing the flavor. (The French call the transformation *mortification*.) After three or four weeks of dry aging, a layer of black mold spores grows on the outer cap of fat. That is the sign the meat is in excellent condition — ready to eat. It has lost 10 to 15 percent of its weight through drying. In addition, perhaps 10 percent of the spoiled surface must be cut away. Despite the general trend toward dividing the meat into the major cuts at the packing house, vacuum-sealing it there in plastic, and shipping it in cardboard boxes, high-quality quarters can still be seen hanging in walk-in coolers behind some meat counters.

Meat is sometimes aged inside the plastic package — without loss of weight, without microbial growth on the surface, and without waste due to spoilage. Visually there is no change. The result is as tender as dry-aged meat, but unfortunately the flavor is not the same. Beneath the plastic, lactic acid–producing bacteria, the same ones that are active in cheese-making, are at work. When the package is first opened, there is a sour smell. (If the process goes too far the smell is very sour.) The difference in flavor is distinct: dry-aged meat tastes better. I once asked an older chef from France about aging in plastic. He immediately responded, "Bullshit!"

Aged beef is sometimes described as more intensely "beefy" and "nutty"; it has been compared to roasted pecans. Among other changes, the fat has begun to turn rancid, a definite component of the aged flavor. People who aren't familiar with the taste of well-aged beef don't always like it, but in cattle country some people have nearly made a cult out of aging prime beef.

For unadorned foods like roast beef to succeed, the quality of the ingredients must be high and close attention must be paid in cooking. Two reasons for roasting beef on the ribs are that when those bones are cut away beforehand, more meat fibers are cut, so more juices are lost during roasting, and that the ribs offer more protection to the meat. A boneless rib-eye roast is drier. Then, too, there is something almost necessary about the appearance of whole ribs at the table.

13

Eggs

The egg of nearly every creature is or has been eaten somewhere in the world. For many centuries, the favorite has been the egg of the chicken, not least because it could be readily had from a tame animal in the dooryard.

In a less populous, less affluent European past the eggs of wild birds were commonly gathered. The New World was so rich in fish and game that we don't seem to have taken the trouble to stalk nests. These days quail eggs, which frequently accompany quail dishes, are a byproduct of raising quail. Among wild birds, the eggs of the lapwing became fashionable in France, partly due to the praise of Brillat-Savarin. Plover eggs, like turtle eggs, had cachet in England for a long time. Also in England, seagull eggs were gathered from nests into the twentieth century. One of my favorite writers, Dorothy Hartley, wrote in *Food in England:* "The seabird eggs sold around the coast were sometimes fishy in taste (like the penguin eggs sold at the Cape), but were usually eaten after so many herrings, so that the flavour passed unnoticed. I had gulls' eggs in Durness, served on hot buttered toast spread with bloater [partially cured herring] paste. They were very good."

Next most popular after chicken eggs are duck eggs. A few years ago in the spring, I was given half a dozen of them. Some shells were dirty white and others, light blue. Duck eggs are larger than chicken eggs, with extra-large yolks that leave little room for whites. The raw egg has the same faint, slightly gamy odor as raw duck flesh, although the taste is mild enough to go undetected in caramel custard, where duck eggs behave more or less as chicken eggs. But the whites make poor foams: there are no duck-egg soufflés. The cooked white, at least of the ones I had, was whiter than that of a chicken egg. Third most popular in the West are goose eggs. I asked after them last spring, but I was already too late. They are larger still than a duck egg and are said to have a similarly enlarged yolk and a more pronounced taste.

The chicken egg has the most practical balance of white and yolk and is the most convenient size, but I think it was primarily the flavor that caused the chicken above all other birds to be tamed and bred to produce eggs. The chicken egg tastes rich, but the flavor is unattached to a specific animal, just as chicken flesh was a relatively neutral canvas for the grand chef's palette, making it prized until mass production deprived the tender plump chicken of its specialness and made its refinement mundane. As chicken flesh is delicate compared with red meat, so are chicken eggs compared with gamier ones. But, as happened with the flesh, industrial-scale production has cheapened the egg in our eyes. To the extent that eggs remain within the bounds of high-style food in the United States, it is due to the unique froth produced by the whites in dishes such as mousses and soufflés and somewhat to the unctuousness of the yolk in sauces and custards. Yet, the taste of well-produced egg, all by itself, is delicious.

The bird that, with a little help from elsewhere, is the original of our chicken is *Gallus gallus*, the wild jungle fowl that is still found in India and Southeast Asia. Like most domesticated hens, most wild jungle fowl lay white eggs. (The color of a domestic chicken egg, of course, depends on the breed and tells nothing at all about quality.) The bird was first tamed perhaps five thousand years ago. Persians learned of the birds in India, and apparently they taught the Greeks. In Rome, the chicken was still more esteemed and was differentiated into several breeds. Like so many other culinary developments, the chicken spread up the Italian peninsula and into northern Europe (although there is a suspicion that a northern European chicken may have at the same time spread southward). Apparently some credit for developing the domesticated chicken belongs to ancient Egypt as well.

By the late nineteenth century, Americans and Europeans were fervently breeding chickens. The old poultry books dwell lovingly on the breeds, their origins, and precise traits. The coloration that was achieved was striking. Almost all the breeds bear place-names plus a reference to color — white, buff, black, silver, golden, blue, red, barred (black and white). Among the old breeds are Plymouth Rock (a Connecticut hybrid from the 1860s), Orpington (from Kent, England; the Black were first), Wyandotte (disputed origin), Rhode Island Red (the local chicken that was developed in the state in the mid-1800s and comes only in red), Leghorns (originally from Italy), Cochin (came to England from China in 1835), Brahma, Hamburg, Minorca, and so on.

Today, from the 30 or so eggs laid in a year by wild *Gallus gallus* hens, *Gallus domesticus* hens have been induced to lay 250 eggs and more. The old general-purpose meat-and-egg chicken is now an amateur's bird. Separate chickens for intensive meat or egg production have been synthesized from some of the old breeds to the point where current textbooks don't speak of breeds but strains and numbers. The niceties of the old breeds are irrelevant to demands for meatier birds, more productive layers, calm chickens for factory cages, and always for meat birds with *white* plumage, so pinfeathers missed in plucking don't show unpleasantly black. Anyway, when it comes to quality in eggs, the particular breed doesn't seem to matter. What is important is the way the hens are raised.

Except during a recent shortage when a fox ate most of his pullets, I usually buy my eggs from a neighbor who raises various animals, including a milk cow. The chickens are fed conventionally, but the eggs are fresher than supermarket eggs, with firmer yolks and whites. The yolks also have a strong yellow color. I used to get eggs with very uncommercial qualities from a friend who lives high on the cold side of a hill. The shells were thick, and some coming from Araucana hens were blue; notably firm whites surrounded striking firm, orange yolks. My friend fed them standard chicken pellets, but the birds roamed outdoors, where they supplemented the commercial feed with the more traditional miscellany of green plants, seeds, worms, and insects. Green plants help to give color to the yolks. Unfortunately, my friend sold his chickens. But there are one or two other sources close by, with eggs nearly like the ones from that cold hill.

Some of the people connected with commercial egg raising deny that there can be superior quality in eggs from these small flocks — call them free-range or what you will. They say, oh, those eggs are just fresher. Nonsense. I've kept my neighbor's small-flock eggs for weeks, and then they still look different from store eggs, and the robust texture of the raw egg still carries over into a firmer, lighter omelette or whatever is made. This is true to the point that in some preparations firmness is a disadvantage or fewer eggs are required. The quality is maintained even in winter, when the hens get neither grass nor garden scraps and are mostly cooped up. I can only guess that summer diet and exercise help tide the hens over the winter. And I assume that much of the quality results from not forcing the hens to produce at the extreme limits of their abilities through artificial lighting, rigid confinement, controlled temperature, additives to feed, occasional drugs, breeding to a rarefied state, and so on. Still, the most important influence on egg quality is the kind of food. (Escoffier: "I have made several experiments in this field; three boiled eggs have each had a different taste, the reason being that the hens which laid them were let loose and fed upon different foods.")

Here's the opinion of Bill Murphy, a farmer who also teaches pasture management at the University of Vermont and has a reputation that extends far beyond the state. In *Greener Pastures on Your Side of the Fence* (1987), he writes,

Most people don't even know what good chicken or eggs taste like, because in their lifetimes they haven't eaten any that were produced on pasture. I know that the things produced in confinement are called chickens and eggs, but that's where the similarity ends. You can do it another way.

As he explains,

Poultry produced on pasture? Of course! That's the way it is still done on small diversified farms, and that's the way it used to be done on all farms before this latest trend toward confinement feeding of all livestock began. Confinement feeding of livestock was encouraged by the availability of inexpensive grains. Economically, I suppose that made sense, but from the viewpoints of ecology, soil erosion, food quality, and responsibility for the world community, it never makes any sense to feed grain to livestock unnecessarily. Grain never really is cheap to produce in terms of energy used and costs of soil nutrients and erosion.

One wonders whether pasture, compared with a grain diet, may also benefit the fats and healthfulness of eggs. Unfortunately, it isn't only fear of cholesterol and calories — at about eighty calories apiece eggs aren't too bad — that makes people wary of eggs. (Some people believe that an egg fertilized by a cock overcomes some of the cholesterol problem, but, as far as I can learn, fertilized eggs have neither a nutritional nor a culinary advantage.) More recently we have learned there can be salmonella in the eggs as well as in the meat of chickens. Only a tiny percentage of eggs is contaminated, and the problem may always have existed, since like other forms of microlife salmonella pervade our environment on a low level. Or the problem may have been aggravated by mass production. As for me, on the wholly unsubstantiated suspicion that the dooryard eggs I buy may be healthier and safer, I still use an occasional raw eggs and I don't cook my eggs any harder than I like.

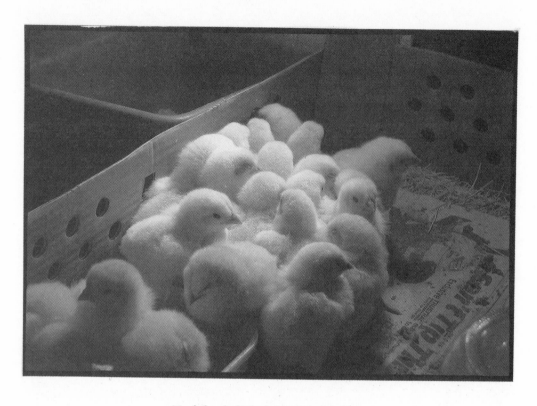

Newly hatched Rhode Island Red chicks at
Lovejoy Brook Farm. Andover, Vermont, 2003.

Without a raw egg, there can be no mayonnaise, since the supermarket product has almost nothing to do with the true olive oil-yolk-mustard-lemon sauce. And without a lightly cooked egg, there are no poached eggs to make wonderful combinations of yolk and sauce, no delicate omelettes, no custard sauces. The kind of risk we choose is cultural. By some American standards, Europeans accept unreasonable risk in consuming young raw-milk cheeses. The Japanese accept risk in the way they eat fish. Americans insist on a nearly fail-safe food supply, but on the highway we accept a huge risk in exchange for mobility.

In the 1960 edition of the *Larousse gastronomique*, which I like for its frank Gallic prejudices and more complete entries than the edition that followed, there are almost twenty pages of egg recipes, as many as thirty per page. The newer edition contains fewer than six pages of recipes, set in larger type next to a larger number of pictures. It is true that many of the old recipes are forgettable reshufflings of ingredients, but they recall the former importance of the egg. I can't remember ever seeing an egg as the main point of a dish on a dinner menu in an ambitious American restaurant. We seem to have forgotten the aesthetic pleasure of the egg; we find it distasteful by association.

Yet eggs can take an extraordinary variety of forms and can display textures that emphasize different aspects of flavor. Cooking sets eggs tenderly to firmly in the obvious manifestations of soft-to hard-boiled, baked, poached, and custard. Combined in various preparations and swollen by heat, they puff omelettes, help to raise brioche, bubble Yorkshire pudding (popovers, crêpes, and *clafoutis* all come from the same batter), and, dramatically, blow up *pâte à choux* into cream puffs. The beaten whites structure soufflés, mousses, meringue, and certain cakes. Whites make crisp cookies. Whole eggs beaten into foam along with sugar raise a *génoise*, the classic cake that predates baking soda and powder (and has a firmer texture than powder-leavened cakes). And egg yolks assist the water-oil emulsion in mayonnaise and lemon curd, as they bind and thicken other sauces.

An egg gathered from the henhouse is sometimes dirty with droppings and perhaps has clinging straw or down. The porous shell has a natural wax, which commercially is replaced with oil after the eggs are washed. (To store eggs for a long time, people used to dip them in paraffin to seal them completely.) The shell of an egg is good protection, but a cracked egg may quickly spoil and should be thrown out. The calcium-rich shells make good compost; people who keep chickens feed the shells back to strengthen future shells. Under the shell is the thin double skin that can be troublesome to peel, and between its two layers at the wide end is the air space, which grows larger as the egg ages and loses moisture. (A way to tell something about freshness is to see how high an egg floats in water: the lower it is, the fresher.) Most of the white is in one viscous layer, but altogether it is divided into four layers, alternately thick (viscous) and thin. A portion of thick white is twisted at each end into the chalazae that anchor the yolk in the otherwise loose white. (Cooking fully fixes the movable yolk, which is why a boiled egg spins smoothly and a raw egg wobbles.) All of the fat and much of the vitamins and iron are in the yolk. A blood spot on a yolk comes from a biological accident in the hen; if you find one in a commercial egg that is because it was missed when the egg was candled.

A very fresh egg broken onto a plate sits high and firm with a cloudy white. As the white grows older, it becomes clear and increasingly liquid. Together yolk and white are about three-quarters water, but more of the water is in the white; the yolk thins gradually as, with the passage of time, water passes into it from the white. The weak, swollen yolk of an older egg is more liable to break. And its runny white rapidly spreads, making it unsuitable for a neat poached egg. The difference between eggs graded AA and A is a negligible degree of freshness. It is claimed that under refrigeration supermarket eggs will last four to five weeks beyond the date on the carton.

Before refrigeration, freshness was the first point of egg quality. Some very good old cookbooks suggest that an egg to be soft-boiled and served plain should be one laid that morning or at least within the last twenty-four hours. (One of those cookbook writers is Madame Saint-Ange. Her wonderful book of bourgeois cooking, first published in the 1920s and still in print as *La Cuisine de Madame Saint-Ange,* is a model for all who have followed and tried to explain both how-to and why. She defined an *œuf à la coque* as having the white thickened into cream without any of it actually solidified and as having the yolk very hot. The same textural concern occurs with French scrambled eggs, which are nearly custard.) Each egg first used to be broken into a small dish before it was added to anything else, in case it was spoiled, to avoid ruining the whole. In the market, winter eggs were suspect, since they were likely to have been stored.

An egg is supposed to age in one day at room temperature as much as it does in a week in a refrigerator. In the refrigerator, eggs should be kept in a closed container because they absorb odors as well as lose moisture. However, a room temperature egg makes any egg preparation lighter, and the yolk combines more easily with other liquids, even with its own white. Cold eggs can be quickly warmed in a bowl of hot water.

Custard in its ideal state is lovely, at once velvety, light, rich, smooth, and delicate. With its luxury of cream and elegant taste, it evokes for me all that is classically French. And yet, add a nutmeg-flecked skin, and it is very close to homely, soothing American "baked" custard. Custard belongs to many cuisines.

I have a small critical passion for custard, particularly a poached custard. The suave texture of a carefully poached custard and its delicate poise on unmolding bear no resemblance to its black-sheep relative, the overcooked custard. This commonplace misery is marked by a release of watery liquid, a nearly rubbery resistance to the spoon, and a haze of tiny bubbles. Another troublemaker, once all too frequent, is the restaurant *crème caramel* that relies on flour to bind the product together despite overcooking and that waits in the cooler for days before being dumped in a chilly lump on a plate and presented to the diner. In that case, you search in vain for a melting lightness on the tongue. Lately in a better style, custard has returned to the menus of fashionable American restaurants.

Custard is nothing more than a cup of liquid set by an egg with the aid of mild heat. Careful cooking produces a perfectly voluptuous texture, achieved by a balance between over- and undercooking. The cook uses a low oven, placing the dish in a larger pan of hot water, a bain-marie, to poach the mixture gently in water that must never boil, and covering the top to avoid a skin (although some people like the skin). The water bath is superfluous when a custard is protected by pastry, as in a savory quiche or a raisin custard pie. Impatient cooks may choose a higher, faster heat and try to pull the pan out of the oven before the damage is done, but low heat gives the novice or busy cook a much wider margin in which to act and to my taste produces a finer result.

An experienced eye recognizes doneness by the response of the custard to a small shake of the pan. At that point, in the old home test, a knife inserted in the center comes out clean. But there is no single perfect texture; the rule of one egg to one cup of liquid is there to be violated. Nearly every recipe is enriched by an additional yolk for every whole egg and often quantities vary greatly. (A refined touch is to strain out the albuminous chalazae clinging to the yolk.) A custard to be served in its cooking vessel should be notably tender from extra egg yolks, but a custard to be unmolded must be made firmer by a higher proportion of white and a little more cooking.

Milk and cream are the liquids that bind best with the egg. Here in Vermont at home, my ideal is a custard of farm eggs and unpasteurized Jersey cream served with maple syrup. In restaurants, the familiar and classical presentation was often *crème caramel renversée*, which for some still brings to mind the dowdiest old-fashioned hotel food and stands almost as a symbol of it. But custard was always at ease in a finer context.

Properly prepared, it has a gracefully unaffected presence that is one of the happiest conclusions to a meal. The crunch of a simple cookie is the only counterpoint needed. Good fresh dairy flavors of milk and eggs, slightly assisted by a nuance of vanilla, stand on their own. Or they willingly lend themselves to the flavor of fruit, especially lemon and orange, or to the obvious caramel, nuts, coffee, chocolate, and occasionally to something more exotic.

Taking texture and chemistry to an extreme, you can combine fine chocolate with egg yolks and heavy cream so that custard thickens but won't set at all in a normal sense. At room temperature, the intensity of chocolate flavor and the gorgeously spoonable consistency satisfy an appetite for chocolate through a serving so small that it paradoxically suggests lightness. This dessert is, of course, *petits pots de crème au chocolat*.

The word *custard*, according to the *Oxford English Dictionary*, is an alteration of *crustade* that first occurred at least five hundred years ago, when the word began to lose its clear reference to the pastry container in which it had been cooked. In the first half of the twentieth century, however, the teaching chef Henri-Paul Pellaprat still cited the French *croustade* as meaning crisp pastry enclosing a savory cream filling. And today the Italian *crostata*, a dessert custard in a pie crust, adheres to its linguistic origins.

Outside a crust, custard's delicacy of flavor, texture, and form are particularly suited to a light, modern style of cooking. You can always substitute low-fat milk for cream (and vice versa).

There is conflicting advice as to whether egg whites, in order to whip into higher, lighter foam, should come from fresh or older eggs. On this I trust Rose Levy Beranbaum, who concludes in *The Cake Bible* (1988), "It's six of one, half a dozen of the other. Fresh whites are thicker so they take longer to beat. The resulting foam has less volume but more stability and loses less volume when folded into other ingredients. Older whites are thinner so they beat more quickly and yield greater but less stable volume. When folded into other ingredients they lose the extra volume." It makes no difference.

Beating egg whites not only adds air but alters the protein of the white in such a way that it gives the foam strength — or it would be as weak as soap bubbles. The presence of even a tiny amount of yolk or other fat interferes with the developing structure of protein and prevents the egg whites from expanding as much as they should. Harold McGee in *On Food and Cooking* (1984) says the whites can increase in volume by up to eight times. He explains that the foam is sturdiest just before it reaches its point of greatest volume (stiff peaks), so it is best to stop just short of that. Then if you draw the whisk straight up from the bowl and turn it upside down, the whites hold a nearly vertical point. If you turn the bowl upside down, the whites remain securely in place (though they may slide out of glass). And if you set a whole egg in its shell on the foam, it will support the weight. This foam is also capable of holding, without completely collapsing, fats that are gently folded in. But left alone in the bowl, the beaten foam quickly sets up and then begins to separate and lose liquid; after that, when stirred the foam becomes grainy and deflates, as if overbeaten. So fold in ingredients promptly as well as gently.

Three added substances reinforce the foam and make it more difficult to overbeat. Beating in the traditional copper bowl binds a minute quantity of copper to the egg whites and produces a reassuringly stable foam. The copper bowl should be deeper than a perfect hemisphere, so bits of egg white aren't flung out. The bowl is cleaned first by wiping it with salt and either lemon or vinegar to eliminate grease and verdigris; it is dried with a perfectly clean towel. I enjoy whipping egg whites in copper, but you can get the same result in another kind of bowl by adding a teaspoon of cream of tartar to a cup of egg white. For dessert purposes, sugar added to the beaten whites interacts with the water to prevent the foam from separating, enabling it to hold for a considerable time. But adding sugar at the start dilutes the protein, delaying and reducing the quantity of foam. A little sugar added gradually after almost all the volume has been achieved ensures a stable foam; a lot of sugar makes a stable thick one.

When beating egg whites, start slowly, increase speed, and, if you have to stop at all, stop only momentarily. A strong arm and a balloon whisk large enough to keep the whole quantity moving produce lighter results than a small electric beater does, although a Kitchen-Aid is equal to the task. French cookbooks and their American progeny tell you to add salt when the whites begin to froth, but salt very slightly weakens the foam, and when it isn't needed as seasoning it should be left out.

A soufflé base should be roughly the same consistency as the beaten whites, that is, pourably thick but not so liquid that it will settle to the bottom of the mold. It is safest to bake a soufflé immediately, but the filled and ready mold will wait for an hour or two. And a base and foam that are sufficiently firm and well matched in consistency have been known to wait overnight in the refrigerator before baking perfectly well the next day.

It is a myth that soufflés are susceptible to collapse in the oven. But I do prefer a soufflé that is light and airy enough that it will collapse shortly after it comes out of the oven. The rise is achieved by rapid baking at about 400 degrees Fahrenheit. It will dry from overcooking unless it is taken from the oven when its center is still flowing (though we are told it may be risky to eat). The center continues to cook even as the soufflé is served, which must be done immediately, before the collapse.

A hint of sulfur belongs to the flavor of a cooked egg, but an overcooked hard-boiled egg releases a sulfurous gas from the white that in turn gives a grayish cast to the outside of the yolk. Prompt peeling minimizes the sulfur smell in a hard-boiled egg. To fully hard-boil eggs: put them in cold water and bring them to a boil, boil one minute, then leave them, covered, off the heat for ten minutes. Largely for moister texture, the French prefer the yolk of a "hard-cooked" egg to be slightly soft, or *mollet*; for the set but still-tender yolks of *œufs mollets*, remove the eggs after six to seven minutes. It is true that an older egg peels more easily than a very fresh one and that it helps to plunge the hot egg into cold water before starting to peel.

The flavor of an omelette, apart from its tender, light texture due to an agile wrist (not mine) and high heat, is compounded of plenty of good butter that is first lightly browned in the hot pan. The outside of the omelette should begin to show brown while the inside retains a trace of liquid.

The usual opinion is that eggs mar wine. In the title essay of her *An Omelette and a Glass of Wine*, Elizabeth David writes that "although there are those who maintain that wine and egg dishes don't go together I must say I do regard a glass or two of wine as not, obviously, essential but at least as an enormous enhancement of the enjoyment of a well-cooked omelette.... But we are not in any case considering the great occasion menu but the almost primitive and elemental meal evoked by the words: 'Let's just have an omelette and a glass of wine.'" (She adds, "Perhaps first a slice of home-made pâté and a few olives, afterwards a fresh salad and a piece of ripe creamy cheese or some fresh figs or strawberries.") This glass of wine will almost certainly be white, just possibly pink. With a more involved egg dish dominated by other nonegg ingredients, red wine may be the thing, depending on what those ingredients are.

Certainly, eggs are altogether undervalued these days, especially as a first course (where they can be a medium for vegetables, cheese, fish) — prelude to simple lean meat or fish, roasted or grilled.... But I don't know that eggs will come into favor again soon. There are plenty of other good things to eat, though none comes near to being a substitute for the egg.

14

A Multiplicity of Apples

Possibly, the best apple I ever ate was a Wealthy that I picked one cool, sunny September day some years ago from the last living branch of an old tree in an abandoned farm orchard. Not many orchardists would be impressed by my "best" claims for a Wealthy. Apple people and apple books usually rate it slightly below the top varieties. Yet the deep roots of the dying tree may have concentrated an exceptional store of energy into the final display of fruit (the tree was dead the next year), and if so, the Wealthy I ate was far above the usual run. I recall that that was a good year for apples, perhaps especially for Wealthy. And it was the kind of fine day on a hilltop that opened the senses; so often one is distracted and doesn't really taste things. And, of course, things remembered are almost always better.

Apple flavor is a complicated, contentious matter. Almost before you begin to speak about varieties, some orchardists will warn you that there's no such thing as a best apple. Even so, variety is the most important factor in apple flavor. Anyone's opinion as to the best variety is not only a question of preference but of chance. What apple varieties have you tasted and which were in top form? Was the apple you ate underripe, perfectly mature, or settling into a soft, flat decline? Not every apple on the tree ripens at once, and for any variety a few days or a week makes a difference. Some evolve very rapidly. Apple notions vary according to where you have lived or traveled in apple season. What do you call delicious in an apple? My own count of varieties has been boosted by the many nameless ones I've collected along back roads. Alerted by windfalls lying in a dusty semicircle at the edge of the road, I pull over, or I tromp through an overgrown field to reach some unkempt tree — far from a house and so unclaimed, I hope. Such apples are most of the time disappointing, but they are an education in the near-infinite diversity of apple flavor.

Each apple seed contains countless genetic possibilities, which are continually expressed in the seedlings that sprout readily from seed of apples tossed or fallen on the ground (popping up like wildflowers in unmown fields). The various species that make up our modern apples are impossible to sort out, since even in the wild they hybridized and mutated for thousands of years before they were taken into cultivation. But our mongrel apples are essentially *Malus pumila*, which spread through Europe from the Caucasus and Turkestan, where the species still grows wild. There, along with small sour apples, some wild trees occur with good-sized edible fruit comparable in quality to cultivated fruit. The ancients were fond of apples; in the first century AD Pliny mentions twenty-three varieties. One apple that is reputed to survive from classical times is the Api, or Lady Apple, a lovely small, flat, red apple that is still a specialty in the United States around Christmas. The Romans probably introduced the first cultivated apples to England, and the original American apples came largely from England, although English apple stock was enriched at various times from the Continent. Notably, Richard Harris, fruiterer to Henry VIII, imported apple varieties from France and Holland to plant a hundred acres of apple and cherry trees. The first apple trees on the American continent were probably all grown from seeds, perhaps saved from Dutch and English apples eaten on board ship, though scions of some named European varieties were imported later. The apple's genetic variability easily gave rise to varieties adapted to many specific conditions around the world. Most Old World varieties didn't fare well in North America and were abandoned. North America's native apples are crabs, and it is unclear how they got here.

Unless an apple blossom is protected from insect-borne pollen and intentionally fertilized with selected pollen — as is done today with the tip of a camel's-hair brush — the second parent can only be guessed at. In the open, each seed in an apple may have been fertilized by a different parent, and in any case each produces a tree with a unique combination of characteristics. Without the techniques of grafting (or of rooting a branch), each tree in the world would constitute its own distinct variety.

The Wealthy arose from an unusually intent search by one man, but the method was the same as for more carelessly bred apples of the same period. The first Wealthy tree grew from seed planted by Peter Gideon in Minnesota in the 1860s. The seed came from an open-pollinated Cherry Crab. For ten years Peter Gideon planted enough seed to grow a thousand trees each year, so as to select only the finest trees. Then, in the winter of the tenth year, extreme cold killed all his trees and, he wrote, "all hope of apple culture in Minnesota was gone. I at once resolved to leave the State, and so informed the family, at which they all rejoiced. [But] I went to bed after coming to this decision, and was impressed to try once again, and wrote to Maine for seeds and cions [sic]. . . . I spent what little money I had in getting this Maine stock, and denied myself the suit of clothes I needed sorely, to start again." His method was the old one of simply planting several different varieties close together and relying on nature to distribute the pollen randomly among them. Of all the seeds that Peter Gideon planted, the best fruit came from the cold-tolerant tree we know today; Wealthy was the given name of his wife. This history, along with that of hundreds of other apples, is recorded in *Apples of New York*, by S.A. Beach of the Geneva Experiment Station, a two-volume work published in 1905 that is still a standard reference. It is so thorough it might as well have been called *Apples of the United States*. (The book offers a history in brief and directs you to Gideon's own account.) The Wealthy reached the height of its commercial success in the 1910s and 1920s when it was briefly overplanted and the market was swamped. Today it is commercially unimportant and declining still further. It is a tart apple, pleasant eating, but not very different from a lot of other northern apples.

I am prejudiced toward tart apples. Though I grew up in Maryland, I have nearly always had a cold-climate attitude toward apples. I associate them with the first cool days of late summer or with bracing days in autumn, when snow is a not-too-distant possibility. What this weather requires are tart Gravensteins, Duchesses, Northern Spies, McIntoshes, Macouns, Fameuses, at a pinch Cortlands — all of them with a satisfying tang when freshly picked. A few years ago I drove out into the Virginia countryside in October to buy fruit and sweet cider and found that Virginia cider and apples, at least the ones I came across, were bland compared with New England ones. Expecting a near jolt of tartness, I found it hard to be sure I was tasting much of anything. But I know there are more interesting apples than the ones I met; I was entirely too close to the mainstream. Almost two-thirds of Virginia's crop are either the insipid Delicious or, what I find worse, Golden Delicious — the living essence of a canned apple: flavor without dimension, sweetness without backbone. Every apple requires at least a hint of brisk acid. For one, I should have been looking for an Albemarle Pippin, discovered before 1750 in Newtown (now Flushing), Long Island, and also known as Green or Yellow Newtown.

Perhaps eight thousand apple varieties exist in the world today (a number of them closely related), and probably most people haven't tasted even a dozen. There was a time when I hadn't tasted many myself, and I was easily impressed. Real apple fanciers tend to dismiss McIntosh out of hand. Macoun, an eighty-year-old combination of McIntosh and Jersey Black, would beat it in any flavor competition. Happily unaware of this, for a long time before I ate that Wealthy I thought of a certain McIntosh as the best apple I ever ate. I picked it at the peak of its October maturity from a tree in a commercial orchard. Strictly speaking, I stole it. The orchard was in that cold part of New York and northern New England sometimes called

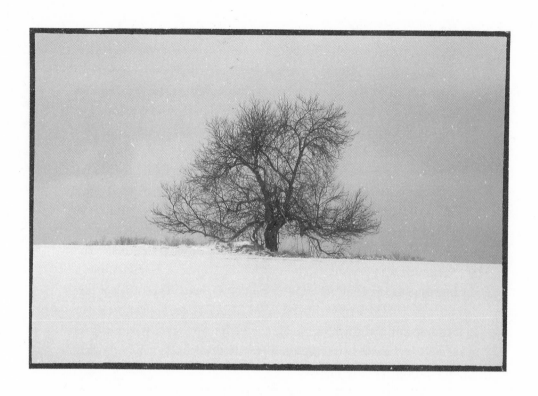

*Old apple tree of unknown variety
during spring melt. Groton, Vermont, 2004.*

"McIntosh country." As I remember it, this Mac had archetypal McIntosh qualities — simultaneous strong tartness and sweetness, an almost-tough skin bursting over soft juicy flesh, and the distinctive McIntosh flavor sometimes called vinous. But, as any orchardist will tell you, "A stolen apple always tastes better." And certainly I've tasted more and better apples since.

The McIntosh was discovered by John McIntosh in about 1811 as a seedling tree in a stand of second growth in Dundas County, Ontario. It was transplanted next to the house. With his find, John McIntosh and his descendants turned nursery growers, but it took almost a hundred years for the variety to become generally known (which was coincidentally about the time the original tree died). The McIntosh was possibly a child of the Fameuse, or Snow Apple, a fine Quebec apple of uncertain antiquity (eighteenth-century or earlier, possibly French) with very white, tender, sweet flesh and a flavor reminiscent of the McIntosh. Or the McIntosh may have come from the Saint Lawrence apple, another variety of unknown early date that is probably from Quebec.

McIntosh country is near the northern limit of apple country. The variety became widespread only following the 1917 freeze, when in the far north for days the temperature remained below −40 degrees Fahrenheit; the apple's spread was further encouraged by the harsh winter of 1933–34, when more tender varieties like Baldwin perished. But even the very hardy McIntosh prefers the temperature-moderating effect of a large body of water.

Joe Costante, apple specialist at the University of Vermont, says that the Lake Champlain valley of Vermont and New York offers "the best conditions for Macs in the world." He credits the influence of the large lake, the soil (loam or clay loam), elevation, latitude, and terrain (hillier than the terrain of Canadian orchards). The cool nights in the fall trigger the formation of red pigment in the skin (from anthocyanins; the same color-climate-ripeness relationship occurs in red grapes). But because of the lake there are no extreme temperatures to damage the blossoms in spring or the ripening fruit in fall, nor is there baking heat in summer. Lake Champlain freezes over only during some winters, and the westerly winds descending from the Adirondacks are compressed as they fall, also making the air warmer. A key to protecting any orchard is air drainage: free downhill air movement through trees planted on a slope. On frosty nights, freezing air moves past the orchards and slides beneath the warm air on the valley floor, which is then sandwiched between the cold above and below. Joe Costante explains, "You have to be detail minded for commercial success." And he runs down a daunting list of necessary care, ending by saying, "And all that can be wiped out by fifteen minutes of hail." His favorite apple? "I still like a Macoun."

The top US apple-growing state by far is Washington, where apples are grown especially in the central area near Yakima and Wenatchee. Second is now Michigan, where apples are concentrated on the leeward side of Lake Michigan (which doesn't freeze). New York has been edged into third place; apples there are grown especially along Lake Ontario and in the Hudson River valley. Other major producers are California, Pennsylvania, Virginia, North Carolina, and West Virginia. On a map of the eastern United States that shows concentrations of apple orchards, you can roughly trace the path of the Appalachians.

France is the largest European producer. Italy is not far behind. (The Soviet Union is the world's largest producer.) The average person in France consumes five times as many apples as the average American, mostly in the fermented form of cider. Two-thirds of the French crop is now Golden Delicious, and Jonagold (a cross of Jonathan with Golden Delicious) is advancing. Among famous old and still-admired French varieties is the Calville Blanc d'Hiver, which goes back to at least 1598, although the Calville is little grown anymore even in France. The United Kingdom is presently a meager producer, but it has a grand apple tradition. The salient feature of British apple growing is the mild island climate, which tempers extremes of hot and cold more than any area in the United States. On the other hand, such American varieties as McIntosh, Melrose, and Yellow Newtown don't ripen properly in England because the climate doesn't offer the necessary combination of bright sunny days and contrasting cold nights. Once, the most popular varieties in each apple-eating country were native ones, but now around the world a significant mixing of varieties has begun.

Today's top American supermarket apples, in order of quantity produced, are Delicious (over 40 percent), Golden Delicious (16 percent, no relative but named after Delicious), McIntosh (7 percent), Granny Smith (6 percent), and Rome Beauty (6 percent). They are not often at their finest in stores, and the names don't bring to mind the romance of apples. Delicious and Golden Delicious are late-nineteenth-century apples that came to prominence in the twentieth century. The promoter of Delicious came up with the name before he found the apple to stick it on. Rome Beauty is a mediocre lingerer that first bore fruit in about the 1840s. Granny Smith is the leading apple in Australia; the original tree (from the seed of an apple thrown out in the yard of Mrs. Thomas Smith of Eastwood, near Sydney) was bearing by 1868. It is a newcomer to North America, and the American-grown examples lately in stores are inferior to the previous imports.

In contrast to the familiar commercial successes, the names on the long list of old apples often seem wonderful: King of Tompkins County, Wolf River, Twenty Ounce, Duchess of Oldenburg, Lady, Mother, Hubbardston Nonsuch, Westfield Seek-no-further, Esopus Spitzenburg, Mammoth Black Twig, Black Gilliflower, Yellow Bellflower, Blue Pearmain, Redstreak, Gooseberry, Chenango Strawberry, Melon, Winter Banana, Tolman Sweet, Vittles and Drink, Sops of Wine, Maiden's Blush.

Almost all these antiques originated in North America and most had some commercial importance in 1900 or earlier. Nursery stock or scions from a collector can still be had. The old names, if not fanciful, were sometimes plainly descriptive. The first Smokehouse grew near William Gibbons's smokehouse in Lancaster County, Pennsylvania. The original Bottle Greening tree (the ripe fruit of a greening is green) contained a hollow where farm workers stored a bottle, presumably of hard cider. But the more popular old varieties suffer from a perplexing number of synonyms. The Hubbardston Nonsuch (Hubbardston, Massachusetts, first recorded in 1832) has been known by two dozen and more variants of the basic name, plus American Blush, Farmer's Profit, and, in France, Nonpareille de Hubbardston and Monstrueuse d'Amérique.

By modern commercial standards, the old varieties often have shortcomings. They may bruise easily, store poorly, be plain-looking or outright ugly; their season may be fleeting; or the trees may bear only a scant crop or tend toward a biennial one. Whatever their other flaws, some of the antiques disappeared from the market because they just didn't taste very good. An orchardist who still has some Wolf River trees told me, "It's probably about the poorest apple I grow." A man who finally cut out his Sops of Wine explained, "I never found anyone who thought it was a good apple."

From the 1600s almost up to the present, the apple was by far the most popular American fruit. It was easily grown and it stored well, some varieties keeping until spring, and the fruit also provided an important beverage. From the time of earliest settlement, every farm except those in the hottest regions had an orchard. Grapes or berries may have been gathered in the wild, but most farms grew few fruits other than apples (and those they did grow were also tree fruits: pears, cherries, plums, peaches). People to whom sugar was a luxury must have liked the bland, old-fashioned kind of apple called a sweeting. Those actually don't contain much sugar, but they almost completely lack acid. One I've tried is Eastman Sweet; it was like eating so much cotton soaked in a faint sugar sauce. The grower said of sweetings, "All they had was sugar. No taste at all." Now that we have a selection of fresh fruits year-round, we eat many fewer apples than we once did.

But most apples used to be grown for fermenting into hard cider.

The qualifying "hard" was unnecessary before Prohibition, when "cider" came to mean sweet cider. In other countries "cider" still denotes the fermented drink. In this country the freshly pressed, murky, sweet juice was once called "sweet apple juice." It wasn't for sale; it was given to children at the time of cider pressing. Many barrels of cider were put up in each household every year. Visitors were offered not coffee, tea, or water but cider. It was *the* common drink.

Early fruit-growing manuals devoted many pages to cider-making, as if it were a branch of horticulture. But most cider can't have been very good. Typical cider orchards were composed of unselected seedling trees, since farmers considered that the apples were merely going into cider. And when a criterion was applied, it was usually sweetness, because sweet apples produced more alcohol. Common practice was to let cattle and swine run in the orchards so they would fatten on sweet windfalls, which was tough on the trees, although the feed was free. Only a few of the very well-to-do grew particular varieties for making excellent cider.

But attention was paid to selecting and propagating superior eating varieties. Roxbury Russet may be the earliest-named American variety (probably early 1600s, Roxbury, Massachusetts). Russeting is the brown-tan, slightly rough texture that appears to a greater or lesser extent in patches on the skin of many varieties. Unfortunately, it came to be considered a defect in the United States, and russeting was tolerated only around an apple's stem, where it can still often be seen. By the 1800s in New England, the search for new varieties nearly ran amok with people naming and propagating hundreds of apples. And probably none was as important to apple growing in cold regions as the four cold-hardy Russian varieties that arrived by way of the Massachusetts Horticultural Society from the London Horticultural Society in 1835: Duchess (of Oldenburg), Tetofsky, Alexander, and Red Astrachan. These were followed in 1870 by another important cold-hardy Russian variety, Yellow Transparent, brought in by the USDA. The five Russian apples, in their seasons, offered exceptionally good flavor. Even so, the leading varieties in

1900 were Baldwin (a chance seedling from Massachusetts, about 1740) in Northern orchards and Ben Davis (origin unknown, perhaps around 1800) in Southern orchards. They were good keepers, but neither was top quality and Ben Davis is now usually judged poor. As to really good varieties, at about that time H.E. Vandeman, a USDA pomologist, wrote that "Grimes [a parent of Golden Delicious] is the very best of the dessert apples, and Esopus Spitzenburg, Yellow Newtown, Roxbury, Fameuse, and Hubbardston are all varieties of great excellence."

Early apples, or summer apples, are favorites when they come in but they aren't as tasty as later ones and they don't keep. Late apples tend to be the best keepers. Although Yellow Transparent was a big improvement over the summer apples that preceded it, it is nonetheless to me a disappointment. Its time is so short that almost the only way to enjoy it is to pick it (slightly underripe) and eat it standing beneath the tree. The old saying about Yellow Transparent is: "Ripe at noon and overripe at twelve o'clock." Two early apples I have enjoyed are Mantet (Manitoba, 1920s) and Irish Peach (Ireland, before 1820). Tart, underripe apples, the first of the year, are often picked for cooking.

Until the early part of the twentieth century, scarcely any new varieties resulted from intentional crosses; nearly all were lucky amateur discoveries made against high odds. Almost every tree was full-sized, or standard, unlike the more easily tended dwarfs and semidwarfs of recent decades, which are produced by grafting standard varieties onto special dwarfing rootstocks. The old trees were tall, gnarled and twisting. Some varieties reached skyward, some were spreading, and some nearly weeping. A few of the huge number of varieties that have been lost over the centuries were considered great in their time. (Two hundred years ago varieties were thought to "run out" — both the original and its grafted offspring were believed to degenerate during the lifetime of the original tree, about a hundred-year span.) But probably most of the American varieties that are now gone were lacking in some essential quality, or they would have been appreciated enough that we would have them still. One can only guess at how many varieties altogether have ever been considered worthy of a name; ten thousand is perhaps a conservative guess.

Feelings about apples run strong not only according to variety but along national and regional lines. H.E. Vandeman wrote in 1906 that the apple "is perhaps grown here [in America] with greater success than anywhere else in the world." By 1979 Fred Lape, in *Apples and Man*, had advanced to an adamant position. He asserted that varieties from the northeastern limit of the United States and adjoining Canada have set "the standard of taste" for almost two hundred years. Like most apple critics, Lape damned mild apples; his chapter devoted to Delicious is titled "O Beautiful Red Sawdust." He approved of Northern Spy (East Bloomfield, New York, after 1800) and Esopus Spitzenburg (Esopus, New York, before 1790). And he declared that "in the northeastern United States and southeastern Canada [the apple] found the warm summers and the cold winters suited to its perfect development ... for always the best-tasting apples have come from the northern end of its ranges at the very limit of easy endurance of cold winters."

But Joan Morgan, in an appreciation of English apples and apple connoisseurs (in *Petits Propos Culinaires* 20), writes that "indeed apples grow better in England than anywhere else in the world." And in a sense she may be right. But it takes a moment to explain why, and she is so confident of her point of view that she doesn't bother to defend it except indirectly. One piece of indirect evidence is that there are almost no American connoisseurs to compare with the English ones of whom she writes. (Like the Romans before them, the Englishmen sliced their apples with bone knives to avoid tainting the flesh with metal.) But the most important evidence, unmentioned by Morgan, is the effect of the ocean-tempered English climate.

One of those English connoisseurs was Edward Bunyard, nurseryman and son of a nurseryman, who was perhaps the greatest pomologist of the twentieth century. He was a professional but in a sense he represents the last flowering of the age of the amateur before the overwhelming drive to mass production. Some of his assessments of fruit varieties are contained in *The Anatomy of Dessert* (1929, a book marred by a slight breeziness). Here, "dessert" means fruit, accompanied by wine. In a preface to the American edition, he notes that apples generally grow better north of what he calls the "Grape zone." He continues, "We owe the peculiar excellence of our English Apples to our moist temperate climate; slow ripening is the secret as it is of good wine. Nearly all the famous vintages of Europe are grown near the northern limit of cultivation." But in North America, along the cold northern rim where summers are not too hot, fall turns into winter too quickly for many slow-ripening English apples.

Beyond climate, says Bunyard, "The right season to eat an apple is a matter of importance; to catch the volatile ethers at their maximum development, and the acids and sugars at their most grateful balance requires knowledge and experiment. Many apples will keep far beyond their period of maximum flavour, and in some this moment is so fleeting that they are hardly worth growing; a week-end away from home might prove disastrous." From Bunyard's standpoint good apples were an indulgence not for everyone: "To have the best fruit you must grow it yourself."

In speaking of apples, men like Bunyard relied on analogies most commonly encountered in descriptions of wine, and today their adjectives are used increasingly by Americans. Those include *rich, aromatic, vinous, nutty, spicy,* and *perfumed.* Tasters detect notes of anise, pineapple, strawberry, musk, and honey; and they refer to what might be called apple essence, though there is no apparent consensus as to what that is. Cox's Orange Pippin (from a seed planted about 1825) has been the most widely grown variety in England and is usually the most highly regarded. It reflects the English preference for perfume and spice in apples. I've tasted some of this, but I offer few opinions because I've met only some English varieties — and then only as grown in America.

Another English connoisseur was Morton Shand. He was primarily a writer about wine and architecture, but he acted sooner than Americans to rescue old apple varieties that were in danger of being lost. He explained in a 1948 lecture to the Royal Horticultural Society: "It is in no sense an exaggeration to say that, except for the world's few really great wines, nothing we eat or drink presents such fascinating diversity of savour within the compass of a single generic type, or affords such rare delight to the epicure." Foremost in his mind, of course, were English apples.

One category of apple met a specific need. As H.V. Taylor explains in *The Orchard and Fruit Garden* (London, 1961), "The Englishman always has had a special fondness for his apples, though the degree of this has changed from time to time. For long periods the apples were eaten in the dessert course of the meal and this called for apples with flavour that would blend with vintage ports, and in consequence those with a 'nutty' flavour such as Egremont Russet, Orleans Reinette, Adam's Pearmain, and the Blenheim Orange were specially favoured. Where no port was used those rich in sugars — King of the Pippins, Ribston Pippin, and Rosemary — were pleasing and renowned."

(As in Bunyard, "dessert" here has the particular narrow meaning of a fruit course following the sweet course at the very end of dinner — unless savouries follow. An English friend explains to me that on the dessert plate is a lace mat, and on that a finger bowl with a sweet-smelling flower or petal floating in it; the guest places mat and bowl to his left before setting to work on the fruit. *Dessert*, from the French *dessert*, comes from *desservir*, "to remove what has been served"; hence, dessert is the final course after all else has been removed.)

Taylor goes on to say that "the fact that all these were lacking in juice and somewhat dry, as measured by present standards, mattered little for there was the port to provide the liquid part. All these apples are still worth eating. Today apples are eaten at any time of the day, between and with any meal, and those with abundant juice have become popular. The 'spicy' flavour is now preferred to the 'nutty' flavour, and especially if associated with an aromatic aroma. These characters are to be found in the Cox's Orange Pippin, the Ellison's Orange, Laxton's Fortune, Laxton's Epicure, and Tydeman's Late Orange, and all these give real pleasure when eaten in their correct season of maturity." The dozen English apples mentioned by Taylor include most of those frequently cited as superior. A notable omission, suitable for growing in America, is Ashmead's Kernel. It is important to understand that many of the spicy and nutty flavors may not appear unless an apple is picked at the correct maturity and then stored for a period.

The emphasis on subtlety raises the question of the right temperature to bring out fully an apple's flavor. Obviously, an apple eaten ripe from the tree is the temperature it is (in the sun, a dark red one can be as warm as soup). Most of the American apple people I've spoken to like an apple right out of refrigeration, so the fruit presents the stimulation of cold and juice and flavor all at once. Cold tends to mute sweetness, while it doesn't affect sourness, so a refrigerated apple is brought into tarter balance. (Someone who likes cold apples may prefer tarter apples than he realizes.) And a cold apple is crisper. The Englishmen writing fifty or more years ago would have their apples at the cool room temperature of a house without central heat. A particularly aromatic apple should be cool enough to be refreshing, but warm enough to taste completely.

All these fine and sometimes rare apple qualities belong to a fruit eaten raw, out of hand (or with a knife on a plate) — *dessert* apples — as opposed to *cooking* apples or, what are truly obscure in America, *cider* (hard cider) apples. No clear line separates cooking varieties from dessert ones, but an apple distinctly for cooking contains significantly more acid. It tastes tarter, though it may actually have as much sugar as another apple, and it requires sweetening. Its acidity provides a punch of interest to replace the fresh fruit flavors that dissipate in the heat of cooking. Baked apple desserts are one of the best and surest complements to Sauternes, as long as the wine is sweeter than the dessert. More humbly, caramel is the flavor most flattering to cooked apples, as in caramel sauce and a well-browned crisp flaky pastry — essentially, a *tarte Tatin* — or a sweet gratin or simply sliced apples sautéed in butter (without sugar, those can accompany pork or game). The ubiquitous flavor of cinnamon, although delicious, distracts from a fine apple.

In America, we rarely differentiate between dessert and cooking apples; most are "dual purpose." And while this simplification may seem like a recent ploy to bamboozle the public (which may suspect that an apple promoted for both purposes is good for neither), in the United States all but a few very acidic or very sweet apples have always been considered dual purpose. This is so much the case that I can't cite a single American cooking apple by name (though I've picked acidic apples for cooking from nameless trees). In England, by far the most common cooking apple has been Bramley's Seedling (about 1810, its original tree reported still healthy in mid-twentieth century), too tart to eat out of hand.

The contemporary American connoisseur and amateur orchardist Robert A. Nitschke has perhaps considered varieties for cooking as carefully as anyone. He cites Red Astrachan, Stearns, and Porter as having flavors that are altered and made more delicious by cooking. And among his other special likes are Ashmead's Kernel, Golden Noble, Northern Spy, King of Tompkins County, Opalescent, Belle de Boskoop (the most famous Dutch apple), and Calville Blanc. Many apples break down in cooking, some almost into fluff. Apples in an advanced state of ripeness collapse more readily; immature apples resist collapse. Apples that hold their shape include Northern Spy, Golden Delicious, Granny Smith, Rhode Island Greening, and Yellow Newtown.

True cider apples scarcely exist in North America. Hard cider is apple wine, and like grape wine it benefits from age. In the seventeenth century it was the wine of Britain, the drink of gentlemen — before it was displaced by wine from France. By some accounts, that was the end of good English cider. Any moderately sweet apple will ferment and produce alcohol, but not just any apple will make good cider. Four qualities are needed: sweetness, acidity, astringency (from tannin), and aroma. The same four — but much less tannin — are found in good sweet cider. For either drink, a blend of fruit is preferred, except in the case of a handful of cider apples, each of which can go it alone. As recently as fifty years ago, the varieties of cider apple in France and England were believed to number in the thousands.

Only about 5 percent of the blossoms on a tree eventually become apples, and many of the excess apples are shed naturally when they are small, in the June drop. After that the fruit on a cultivated tree is thinned by the grower so the remaining apples become larger and better flavored. As with other fruits, sugars and starches are produced in the leaves and stored in the fruit. Ripening is largely stimulated by ethylene gas produced within the fruit. Starch is changed to sugar, acidity diminishes, the hard flesh softens, the white seeds darken to brown, and the mouthpuckering tannins are reduced. (Tannins are a component of all apples, their astringent presence compounding the effect of tartness in some, their near absence reinforcing the vapidity of others.) Finally, the cells connecting the fruit's stem to its branch dry and weaken, and a breeze or a shake of the branch frees the apple and it drops.

By this time the background color of the skin (most apples have a background color) has changed from green to nearly yellow. And for those who know a variety well, that is probably the best guide to ripeness. But anyone can tell something about ripeness by testing how readily the stem separates from the branch. The proper technique is to lift the apple to one side while slightly twisting, to avoid pulling off the spur that will produce future fruit. A blatant signal of ripeness, unless there has been a fierce storm, is a number of windfalls beneath a tree. The apples of some varieties, however, drop before they are ripe, and the apples of a few varieties never drop at all. Big growers take no chances and rely on iodine starch tests to gauge whether enough starch has been converted to sugar. As soon as it has, they must pick rapidly to "beat the drop." Apples bruise fairly easily. For processing they can be picked by mechanical shakers equipped with large fabric catchers, but almost all apples in stores have been picked by hand.

As soon as the fruit is plucked from the tree, ripening speeds up, so the crop is rapidly put into cold storage. More effective than plain cold storage is CA, or controlled-atmosphere storage (low in oxygen and high in carbon dioxide). In either case, temperatures are near freezing and ethylene gas is ventilated. Amateur growers rely on secondhand refrigerators in the basement or improvised fruit cellars.

In certain uncommercial varieties, biological maturity doesn't coincide with maturity for eating. Some of these apples are tastiest when the seeds aren't yet fully dark (by the time they are, the apple is over the hill); others must be picked while their acidity is still high and stored as acidity declines and flavors reveal themselves.

Examining a ripe apple, you see tiny spots dispersed over the skin, more or less prominent according to the variety. These are pores, called lenticels, through which gases are exchanged. Cutting the apple open, in a horizontal cross section you find a ring of spots around the star-shaped core, spots that are vessels for carrying sap from the stem. Marking the pale flesh may be darker areas of water core, where the air spaces between cells are flooded with sweet juice. This delicious phenomenon is unpredictable, and it is a problem for growers because water core turns brown in storage. (For salads, the Cortland, a McIntosh–Ben Davis cross, and the Empire have the advantage that their flesh remains white long after it is exposed to air. They contain very low amounts of phenolic compounds, which include tannins, as well as a particular enzyme, both of which are necessary for browning.) And last, by biting into the apple, you discover not only the flavor but the texture: coarse, fine grained, hard, soft, tender, crisp.

It's no coincidence that the dominant apples in the supermarket are easily identified by color — one wholly red apple, with an unusually long shape and bumpy blossom end (Delicious), one yellow-green (Golden Delicious), one smooth red and green (McIntosh), and one solid green (Granny Smith). Some people think that the next apple to join the group will be a striped yellow and red apple such as Gala (about 1934, New Zealand).

I confess that I have been disappointed by supermarket apples so many times that now I almost never buy an apple in the supermarket to eat raw. And I rarely buy apples there for cooking. I loathe mealy, flat-tasting apples, some losing even their sweetness. To someone who knows apples, a dull whitish bloom on the skin (of Delicious, too) betokens freshness, and the store's wax shine does not. I pick my apples from abandoned trees or I buy them from an orchard; after the season I do without. I've been told that the reason store apples are so bad is that when they are removed from storage to be delivered to supermarkets, they leave refrigeration and they may never be refrigerated again. Weeks may pass before they are eaten. Few supermarkets accept deliveries of local apples. They trade on our memories of apples that once were good. Luckily, there has been a revival of specialty markets, pick-your-own operations, orchard stands, and farmers' markets, where the quality is often high and there is an expanding choice of antique and modern varieties.

I have always believed that superior apples come from venerable full-sized trees with broad root structures to support good fruit. But the experts don't agree with that. And if you are out picking apples, you may like to imagine which is the best apple on a particular tree. It will be one fully exposed to the sun. (Good pruning aims at providing equal light to all.) Of two equally ripe apples on the tree, the redder one probably received more sunshine and has better flavor, though if it is quite red, it may be overripe. And the best apple isn't the largest on the tree or the earliest to ripen; it is a fruit of about average size that ripens midway through the tree's season. It may be the king apple, the largest apple in the center of a truss, or fruit cluster, and usually the only one left in the truss after thinning. Your search may not always be satisfying, since every year isn't ideal for every variety. After the grape, the apple is probably the fruit most susceptible to the effects of vintage.

Almost everyone likes a sweet apple with concentrated flavor; it is only the nuances of flavor and the degree of balancing tartness that are in dispute. If you sample different varieties from one orchard to another, you come to understand that an essential apple virtue is its unexpected variety of flavor, its surprises from apple to apple, tree to tree, and especially from year to year — produced largely by the imperfectly understood influences of soil, cultural practices, climate, and weather. They are filters through which the flavor of each variety is expressed. And, in fact, it is the surprises — the unending variety, not only the high points — that goad you on, that in time are the main reason you go looking in the orchard. As always, for real appreciation you must trust your own taste. You may acknowledge the consensus of connoisseurs, but like each of them (perhaps joining them) you search to please yourself.

Elegy for the Taste of Cream

Until the mid-1980s, the best commercial source of fresh dairy products near me was the Kilfasset Dairy, owned and run by the Kitchel family. Back when I still sometimes drank a glass of milk, I appreciated the superior flavor of Kilfasset whole milk, and the high quality of the cream was unmistakable. A visiting friend from New York, a good cook who loves cream, offered to whip Kilfasset cream and promptly turned it into butter — he was so unused to good cream. After that, he always asked me to bring a quart of cream whenever I traveled down to the city. Unfortunately, the Kilfasset Dairy was sold to a larger dairy, which was sold to a still-larger dairy, which eliminated the old name and the local plant. Each change in ownership brought a deterioration in quality. The last blow, before the name disappeared, was that the dairy began to sell ultrapasteurized heavy cream. The rapid high-heat process (at least 280 degrees Fahrenheit for at least two seconds) alters the cream's taste, its ability to whip, and its texture for whatever purpose. When ultrapasteurization is applied well to fairly good cream, the effects are tolerable — as I admit they are in this case. But more often ultrapasteurized heavy cream is damaged, neutral in flavor at best. Much of it is runny because it has the lowest allowable fat. The effects of ultrapasteurization extend to half-and-half; anyone sensitive to the taste of cream will find an unpleasant difference when this cream is added to coffee. Presumably, that's why the successor to Kilfasset still doesn't ultrapasteurize the half-and-half.

What did the old dairy do differently? The milk came from the family's own large herd of Holsteins and only six or seven other farms. The milk was of excellent quality: it was above average in fat and it tested as very clean. Each state may set its own standards for minimum butterfat, but the standards are generally the federal ones. Whole milk is at least 3.25 percent fat; "light cream" is at least 18 percent fat; "whipping cream" starts at 30 percent; and "heavy cream" starts at 36 percent. Kilfasset heavy cream averaged almost 40 percent. And the cream was pasteurized at a relatively low temperature, about 172 degrees Fahrenheit for fifteen seconds. The milk was homogenized; the heavy cream was not. By reputation, Holsteins produce an anonymous-tasting product, but most Kilfasset milk came from Holsteins, fed and bred for maximum butterfat.

The new, ultrapasteurized version of the cream, by comparison with the old one, is indifferent. The explanation lies partly in the current ultrapasteurization technology. The cream or milk is heated instantly by injecting steam and then a vacuum removes the added water. Various flavors, good and bad, are sucked away at the same time.

The writer Leslie Land pointed out several years ago in an article in *American Wine and Food* (newsletter of the American Institute of Wine and Food) that it is nearly impossible to find excellent cream anywhere in the United States. As she wrote, one reason given for ultrapasteurization is that it compensates for stores' sloppiness about refrigeration (in the old days, the dairies stocked store cases themselves and checked refrigeration temperatures). The dairy companies further excuse their use of ultrapasteurization by blaming consumers for leaving cream out and letting it go sour — and holding the dairy company responsible. But as consumers become even more distant from the freshness that marks quality, won't they learn to abuse ultrapasteurized liquids as well? They don't last forever.

Of course, the primordial tastes of raw milk and cream are alive and well known on every dairy farm. But, unfortunately, few people off the farm can know them.

The taste of cream is mostly the taste of fat. Generally, the more fat in milk or cream, the better it tastes (although people grow used to skim milk and then prefer it to whole milk). What there is of aroma in these fresh liquids is mostly associated with fat. Cream tastes like the milk it comes from, only more so. Except for milk from the odd cow that produces exceptional fat, the order of the solids in milk is: milk sugar (lactose), fats (fatty acids), proteins, and salts (minerals). Fat gives not only flavor but viscous texture. The more fat, the thicker the cream.

By my enthusiasm I don't mean to encourage everyone to eat more fat. (However, for all that is said about avoiding fat, we need to eat some fat, and everyone's tolerance is different.) Certainly one can eat well gastronomically and eat extremely healthy food. Obviously the olive oil in the Mediterranean diet is more conducive to good health than the animal fat that commonly takes its place in the North American diet. Patrick Rance, the great authority on French and British cheeses, notes that the French and Italians eat about three times as much cheese (twelve to fourteen ounces a week) as Americans and have roughly half as much heart disease, despite our reduced smoking and lowered consumption of fat. And he cites several British studies suggesting the key to health is not how much saturated fat you eat but how much polyunsaturated fat. Others have marveled at the same contradictions between American and Continental diets and proposed various explanations for *le paradoxe français*. For the normal person, Patrick Rance advocates a healthy diet marked strongly by variety: meat, cheese, fruits, vegetables, fish, with generous quantities of red wine, garlic, and olive oil.

If cream — or any delicious food that seems to require moderation — is to take its small place in this regimen, it may as well be the best it can be. Or at least we can learn to recognize the best when we can get it.

There is a natural continuum from fresh to ripened cream. Naturally ripened (soured) raw cream is crème fraîche, to use the French word that we now know it by. The parallel in raw milk is curds and whey — or, under the influence of a bacterial culture from a different part of the world, yogurt. To remain sweet for any period of time, cream depends on refrigeration or pasteurization. (The abhorrent taste of sour pasteurized milk comes from decay, not ripening.) Before the days of refrigeration, cream would stay sweet in a cool place for perhaps two days in summer and twice as long in winter. Refrigeration is probably the modern technology that has most benefited the quality of food and drink. Without electricity and refrigeration, the condition of local roads and the distance to the railroad determined whether a farmer's milk went to market as a fresh fluid or was preserved as cheese or well-salted butter (in which case the skim milk was fed to the pigs).

Country people could almost always have sweet, fresh milk and cream, but once upon a time, because most milk and cream had to be transported from the country at an obvious cost of freshness, ripened cream was the form that often came to city-dwellers. Parisians in particular are said to have gained a taste for it. Literally, *crème fraîche* means "fresh cream," a misnomer by our standards because it is ripened; their *crème fleurette* is what we would call fresh. It is crème fraîche that is often intended in French recipes, though the kind of cream is only implicit and sweet "heavy cream" almost always appears in translation.

Pasteurization is a sort of partial sterilization designed to preserve food for a time in exchange for a relatively small loss of flavor. Louis Pasteur developed the technique to solve problems of spoilage in wine, as an outgrowth of his studies of fermentation. He thought the loss of flavor was insignificant, but today no respectable winemaker would agree. And it may be that in milk as in wine, pasteurization destroys flavor esters.

The process definitely alters flavor: pasteurized milk tastes cooked.

This taste is subdivided by dairy professionals into "heated," "cooked," and "scorched" — all degrees of caramel flavor. Something less than "heated" is possible and desirable with low-temperature pasteurization, but distinctly cooked flavors are unavoidable with ultrapasteurization. Even bitterness can result. To be sure, the cream in many dishes is cooked anyway or combined with flavors that overwhelm all but its basic unctuous dairyness. And granted that caramel is delicious. But one would like to enjoy dairy products apart from it; caramel certainly isn't a fresh pastoral flavor.

Other off-flavors can result from such simple things as cows' eating of wild onions or breathing rank odors in a poorly ventilated barn. Rancidity is caused by the enzyme lipase, which attacks fats. Lipase is destroyed by pasteurization but sometimes has a chance to work its harm before that. Most milk is sold in translucent containers, and the most common off-flavor found in milk in stores is caused by light. It shows up after about forty-eight hours in the dairy case, a cardboard or cabbage taste. A man who checks on quality for the state of Vermont told me, "We've raised a generation of kids in the sixties and seventies who think that's the way milk should taste. I don't allow plastic containers in the house." And dairy products are also readily tainted in the refrigerator by odors from other foods such as garlic, since fat molecules are easy for many aromatic compounds to latch on to.

In search of further understanding, I spoke to Sidney Barnard at Penn State University, a respected specialist who has evaluated dairy flavors for many years. The day I spoke to him he had forty-eight milk samples in his refrigerator ready for tasting. If time allows, he and his co-workers first warm the milk to 60 degrees Fahrenheit.

Sidney Barnard is continually tasting raw milk from individual farms, but he is emphatic about the risk: "I drink raw milk all the time. I cannot recommend that anyone else drink it." On rare occasions, undulant fever, tuberculosis, or another disease goes undetected in a cow and her milk goes on the market. Pasteurization eliminates the danger. I asked him about the comparative tastes of raw and pasteurized milk. He doesn't judge one flavor as better than the other; they are "different." He says the milder raw-milk flavors are still present in pasteurized milk, concealed beneath the cooked taste.

Subtle things show against a plain background, and Sidney Barnard appears to be a perceptive critic. He says that it is possible to pasteurize milk and avoid a cooked taste, but only very rarely has he rated milk and found neither a cooked taste nor an off-taste from feed — the other most common shortcoming. He says that to avoid feed flavors the animals should eat nothing, especially not silage, for two to four hours before milking. Contrary to a common impression, cows don't have to eat continuously. (Good small cheesemakers avoid feeding any silage to their cows. For certain European cheeses, the feeding of silage to the cattle is forbidden by law.) When I mention spring pasture, Barnard says that when cows are first put on the lush growth, the milk tastes grassy for ten days to two weeks until the animals adjust. (Rainy weather produces luxuriant grass but diluted milk.) He doesn't concede that any particular feed creates better flavor, only that some cause defects. "Milk with a perfect score is rather bland."

Good milk flavor isn't defined so much by what it is as by what it isn't. This is reflected in the weakness of the common description of "pleasant and slightly sweet." Usually, the flavor is also said to be in some way characteristic. "Cowy" is a word occasionally used, but this more often means that the milk has an off-flavor from an unclean barn (or has a medicinal flavor from acetone, which is a result of ketosis, a physiological problem in the cow).

How long does the fresh raw taste last? Sidney Barnard hesitates to answer at all because he doesn't want to encourage the drinking of raw milk. But then he explains that the answer depends on cleanliness and refrigeration to as low as 35 degrees Fahrenheit. Then the flavor will remain for "a few days and up to a week, if everything is ideal." He confirms that higher fat and other solids give milk and cream the best flavor. "You take the fat out and you don't have that good taste — in any food." Milk from Jerseys and Guernseys, the

Channel Island breeds, has more fat, but besides that it tastes somewhat better than Holstein milk, because the other solids in the "colored cows" are higher as well.

To taste the plain fat, I have made butter from pasteurized Jersey cream that I managed to obtain (as I'll eventually explain). Remembering a simple technique, I shook the cream in a half-full canning jar for about two minutes until it thickened to a slush made of fine fragments of butter in buttermilk. Then I opened the jar and stirred the mixture with a wooden spoon for two or three more minutes until the butter "came" in a thick mass separated from the watery white buttermilk. I poured off the buttermilk and "washed" the butter by stirring it further in several changes of cold water, to rid it of most of the remaining buttermilk, which makes butter spoil more quickly. Last, I kneaded it briefly with a spatula to expel more water. (I drank the sweet buttermilk, which tasted like rich whole milk, not skim.)

Since my butter was made from sweet cream, it was much less flavorful than the butter made from ripened cream, which is the kind you typically buy in the store. ("Sweet butter" is different from "sweet-cream butter.") The taste of my butter was the plain taste of Jersey milk fat. And the color, concentrated from the cream, was so yellow as to make you uneasy if you didn't know the source. But when I tasted the butter side by side with the cream from which it was made, I realized that butterfat alone contains far from the complete flavor and texture of cream that cause us to consume so much of it. Of course, some of the nonfat solids were left behind in the buttermilk, but I think that the biggest difference was the absence of the water that makes foods so much easier to taste.

It is curious that the most productive breeds of dairy cow and dairy sheep were both developed in Friesland, in modern times a province of the Netherlands. The black-and-white Holstein cow, sometimes criticized as a milk factory, is properly the Holstein-Friesian (ironically there is no connection with the region of Holstein), and the most productive dairy sheep is the East Friesland. As our garden and field are largely man-made, so are our domestic animals.

The rich flat fields of well-populated Friesland were historically always expensive and farmers had to be efficient in breeding cattle and in all their work. Each family knew its small herd intimately; barn and house typically shared the same building. As a cultural trait of the region or perhaps because of the economic pressure, all was extremely orderly and scrupulously clean. Equipment was scrubbed multiple times; by two old accounts, there were even curtains on barn windows, and in the stall in winter the cow's tail was kept clean by tying it loosely upright to the ceiling.

Holsteins now make up over 90 percent of US dairy cattle. Only 5 percent of our cows are Jerseys, although the breed is holding its own thanks to the demand for butterfat and protein in cheese and ice cream, supported by improvements in efficiency through identifying top Jersey sires (bulls). Guernseys are well back in third place, followed by Brown Swiss, Ayrshire, and Milking Shorthorn — all of them marginal indeed. One tends to think of rich cream as yellow, and in fact milk from Jerseys and Guernseys is especially yellow from carotene. (Goat's milk contains no carotene at all; its whiteness is obvious in goat's milk cheese.) Beyond the effects of fat and nonfat solids, it is difficult to compare the tastes of different breeds, since it is hard to know what to attribute to individual animals and what derives from soil and methods on different farms. There is no separate milk from different breeds of cattle kept under identical conditions to compare.

I had heard of the small dairy at Hill Farm, not far from me in Marshfield, Vermont, but the farm is up a side road and I had never found the milk in the stores where I shop. Finally, prompted by strong approval of Hill Farm by the head dairy man at the Vermont Department of Agriculture, I paid the farm a visit. Peter Young and his wife, Nancy Everhart, milk a mere eleven cows, all pure Jerseys but one, which is part Brown Swiss; they pasteurize the milk in an old vat pasteurizer that is smaller than any made nowadays in North

America. And in a crisp white refrigerated truck, they deliver the milk themselves to a small group of stores, including a couple of supermarkets. The milk is certified organic and is not homogenized, so it shows a clear line between skim below and cream on top. It is what is called "cream-line" milk.

By acting as their own middlemen — processor and distributor — and by charging a premium for the rarity of organic cream-line milk, Peter and Nancy are able to eke out a farm living with sauerkraut as a winter sideline. Nancy does the pasteurizing using the lowest allowed temperature of 145 degrees Fahrenheit for thirty minutes (cream must be taken 5 degrees higher). Originally, Peter had wanted to sell his milk raw, but he found that it was impossible to obtain liability insurance. On top of that, state regulators now oppose the sale of raw milk.

Hill Farm is about steep enough to call it a sidehill farm, even more aslant than the usual northern New England hill farm. It was not surprising to hear that no cows had been in the fields for nearly forty years before Peter Young came along, although the land slopes southward to catch the sun nicely. In the meantime, the fields had been depleted by haying, before Peter and Nancy built them back up. In June, when I joined a walk to the spring in an upper pasture to check a water line for the cows below, there was a strong honeyed smell from a thick growth of white and red clover in blossom, intermixed with abundant grasses. The cows nuzzled me affectionately.

Peter began the farm. His college concern with world hunger gradually turned to an interest in the domestic food system ("We spend more calories growing food than we get back in the food we've grown"), which he felt in a better position to do something about. He studied sustainable agriculture, and in 1982 through a small inheritance he was able to buy this modest farm. He focuses on the soil, summing up by saying simply that healthy soil grows healthy plants, which produce healthy animals and people. Building up soil is accumulating capital. The chief additions to his soil, besides manure from the barn, are rock powders. He takes the long view. When he spreads his rock phosphate, it will take ten years for all of it to become available to plants. By contrast, the cost of the conventional fertilizer used by the farmer who hays my field is recouped in one season.

At the core of Peter Young and Nancy Everhart's feeding program is a system of intensive rotational grazing. Easily moved electric fencing divides the pastures, and each day the cows are shifted to a new section; what was grazed by the eight milkers one day is grazed by their heifers the next. In this ascending terrain, plowing is an invitation to erosion by rainfall. Except for one badly rough field that required plowing and replanting, and elsewhere some scant overseeding with grasses and clovers, everything that grows now results from the effects of fertilizing and grazing on what was already here. Peter has no plan ever to plow the fields again. He is treating them as permanent grassland as opposed to leys, or temporary pastures, that are periodically plowed up and seeded to chosen grasses and legumes (clovers, vetches, alfalfa) as part of a periodic rotation of crops. He and Nancy do hay some of their fields and other rented land nearby and they make silage. For additional feed in winter, they buy organic corn, soy, and wheat grown in New York State.

Permanent grassland like this eventually arrives at an equilibrium in its variety of species, at least twenty in this part of the country and perhaps many more. Most roots grow in the first three inches of soil, but perennial grasses can reach down ten feet, and the taproot of alfalfa can penetrate thirty feet. The roots of vegetation in drier climates go deeper than those in this moist one. By Peter Young's way of thinking, a pasture is established over as long as a hundred years, as some plants draw minerals from deep in the subsoil, slowly decaying and providing nutrients for shallower-rooted plants. Not only grasses and legumes take hold, but also wildflowers and what might be called herbs of the field, including dandelion, chicory, and plantain, all well liked by cattle.

Observations about pasture are not new. Four centuries ago Gervase Markham, in one of his books about husbandry, observed, "Although the lowe meddowes doe abound in the plenty of grasse, yet the higher grounds even bearth the sweeter grasse, and it is a rule amongst Husbandmen, that the low meddowes do fill, but the high meddowes do feede. The low are for the stable, but the high are for the Cattle, that [grass] which is long will maintaine life, but that which is short will breede milke." High pastures are likely to produce shorter grass because they often are drier and have poorer soil.

A different comparison of ground is made by Patrick Rance, who is probably the clearest explicator of the nature and superiority of farm cheeses. In *The Great British Cheese Book* he points to the similar origins of cheese and wine: "The same species of grape produces completely different wines in different regions, and even in adjacent vineyards of different aspects. So it is with pastures and cheeses." Pierre Androuët's "Letter to My Daughter" in his *Guide du fromage* is good reading for those who love cheese. He writes, "Remember this: all farm cheeses are made from raw milk. They are true to the soil from which they spring." He speaks of the first spring grass, and "then three weeks or a month later the meadows bloom. For me this is the high point of the pasturing season. The fragrance of the opening flowers mingles with the fresh perfume of the tender grass." And, "There are 'growths' [*crus*] of milk just as there are 'growths' of wine."

Scientific studies of traditional dairying scarcely exist in English. The evidence for the validity of old-fashioned distinctions in quality is largely indirect or anecdotal. Again, from Patrick Rance: "Kit Calvert, the most notable veteran of Wensleydale cheese-making, always found the cheese from the higher limestone pastures better than that from the sandier ground near the River Ure. In 1974 when I mentioned the chemists' theory that, given a satisfactory standard of milk, any type of cheese could be made anywhere, he commented, 'That is fast becoming an accepted lie.'" And, "Camembert connoisseurs, according to the late Raoul de May of Louvis, could tell on tasting a farmhouse cheese which side of the hill the milk had come from. The same could be said of Swaledale today: on one small farm I know, sweet cheese comes from the limestone above Oxnop Ghyll, and slightly bitter cheese from the acid peat below."

The French specialist Jean-Claude Le Jaouen probably knows more about goat dairying and goat's-milk cheese-making than anyone else in the world, writes in *La Fabrication du fromage de chèvre fermier*, "The varied flora of natural pastures and the perfumed plants of *maquis* give cheeses a bouquet and a personality directly tied to their *terroir*. This is the source of the notion of a cru of milk, which makes knowledgeable gastronomes seek out cheeses made when pasture is at its peak, *de la pointe de l'herbe*, or during the season of a particular *spécialité originale*. . . . It is precisely due to its personality that a farm cheese can hold its own in the face of industrial production." I have been fortunate in meeting M. Le Jaouen, who clarifies this to say that such a cru would be characteristic of a region, but not of one farm compared to its neighbor. He is little inclined to speculate beyond the scientific studies he is familiar with. The flavors that interest him most are liberated from the fats during the ripening of an aged cheese, well beyond the stage of fresh milk.

Certainly, aged goat's-milk cheese is far afield in taste from fresh cream from a cow. But even in dairy literature in English, you can find a list of "weeds," mostly plants associated with poor pasture, and the unpleasant taints they produce in milk. And the literature also shows that flavors interact, especially in mere traces, reinforcing or obscuring one another — the same substance tasting pleasant or unpleasant according to its concentration. It seems inevitable that for the gourmet, milk and cream must benefit from soil and vegetation with character.

I left Hill Farm with a plastic gallon jug of pasteurized milk. (The translucence of the plastic in which it is sold isn't ideal, but how do you market cream-line milk without showing the cream in either plastic or glass?) All the raw milk had just been pasteurized; I returned on other occasions for that. Peter Young and Nancy Everhart say they aren't especially sensitive to the taste of milk, but they attribute their customers' enthusiasm for it to cleanliness, low-temperature vat pasteurization, and good chilling — on top of the milk's appeal as being local, organic, and unhomogenized. Their care also allows a long shelf life. It is rare that you have a chance to taste the milk or cream of a single farm, since most milk is dumped in with the milk of dozens or hundreds of other farms at a processing plant. Its identity is lost. Hill Farm's rich milk tastes exceptionally good.

A century ago, the only way to separate milk into skim and cream was by gravity and patience. The cream, being lighter, rose to the top, slowly in winter, faster in summer. For many years now centrifugal separators have been used that exploit the same difference in weight between fat and nonfat. In one old separator that I've seen taken apart, the heavier skim milk is thrown to the outside of a series of thin cones contained in a cylinder, while the lighter cream rises up the center, and then the two liquids exit independent spouts.

Clotted, or scalded, cream used to be made in Devonshire and Cornwall (the names this cream is often known by today) after the milk had stood for twelve hours (in summer). The shallow pan was heated gently short of boiling, the slower the better to ensure more cream, until the surface showed thick, wrinkled, and leathery. The cream was cooled and skimmed off the following day. The cooked taste (far beyond pasteurization) was a trait of the cream. Now clotted cream is said to be all made by mechanical separators, except for some made by a rare revivalist or possibly a surviving old-style maker.

To prevent separation, milk is homogenized by forcing it under high pressure through tiny stainless-steel jets, which breaks up the fat globules. Normally, the globules of fat suspended in the lean portion of the milk would tend to clump together and rise, but the fragmented particles in homogenized milk are unable to unite and are too small to rise by themselves. Milk must be pasteurized before it is homogenized, or the broken-up fat will promptly be turned rancid by lipase.

Some people criticize the effects of homogenization, although properly done it is not supposed to change flavor. Changing the fat, however, can definitely change the texture of the cream. Forceful

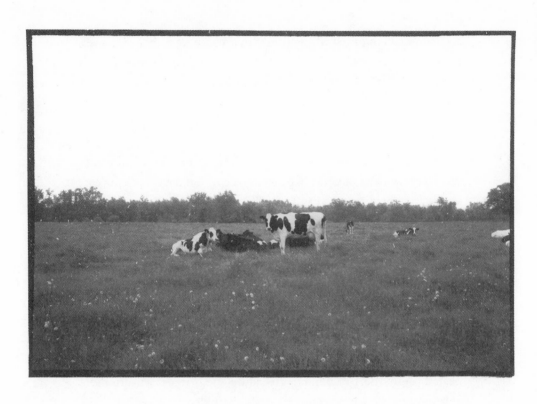

Holstein cows on spring pasture.
Forfar, Ontario, 1996.

pumps are required to push milk through large-scale equipment, and the violent action of a poor pump can break down the structure of the cream. When making whipped cream, the dispersed broken fat globules would prevent the liquid from foaming, as a drop of yolk or other fat does in egg whites. For that reason, the cream for whipping is not homogenized.

Cream roughly doubles in volume during whipping. However, it is the change in texture, not the increase in volume that determines when to stop. Bowl and cream should both be well chilled, or the fat will become too soft to hold the air. (Raw cream whips slightly better than pasteurized.) The intact nature of the fat globules in cream can be seen clearly during home butter-making; as the fat coalesces, the sides of the glass jar become squeaky clean. Only at the end of whipping does the fat begin to break. And only at the end do you sweeten and flavor, as these additions interfere with the developing foam. Powdered sugar is recommended, but it contains cornstarch and I prefer the greater purity of granulated.

Tiny dairies are almost extinct in the United States, but there is a second family farm in Vermont that processes and sells its own dairy products. Jack and Anne Lazor's Butterworks Farm is in Westfield, Vermont, about ten miles from the Quebec border. The herd usually comprises about eighteen cows, all Jerseys. Butterworks Farm produces cream-line milk, yogurt, and cream — no longer any butter. At present, the cream may be the only all-Jersey cream sold in the United States, though several dairies do sell cream-line milk. It was Butterworks cream that I had used to make my own butter. The Lazors' products are pasteurized but not homogenized. Like Hill Farm, Butterworks Farm is certified organic by Vermont Organic Farmers in conjunction with the State of Vermont. Jack Lazor grows most of the grain that carries the cows through the winter, and he aims soon to grow all of it (as he grows the wheat for his family's bread).

As far north as Westfield, the landscape begins to open out, as if someone had loosened the tight folds of the hills and valleys of most of the state. The hills are still high but the wide valleys make room for many more farms. Over the decades, a number of the old Yankees have left and in their place many French have moved down from Quebec. Largely to them Jack Lazor attributes a particular friendliness where he lives.

Not long after I visited Hill Farm, I drove up to Butterworks Farm. I had heard good reports, but I had some misgivings. What is called the cream line in milk is the skim line in cream. Each time I had bought the Lazors' cream in the past, the plastic bottle revealed about half an inch of skim milk in the bottom. More important, at the top was a layer of thick yellow foam full of buttery granules, a problem called "cream plug." This part of the cream would melt into an unpleasant oil slick when I tried it in my coffee (although the cream was really too rich for coffee). But the cream poured carefully out from beneath the plug was deliciously full of flavor, albeit pasteurized. I believe in small farms like the Lazors', but I was puzzled that the concern for quality didn't show in the cream.

Butterworks Farm is a bastion of obsolescent dairying, though with all equipment inspected and approved as necessary by the appropriate bureaucrats. The Lazors still generally move milk from one stage of processing to another in milk cans. But next to the old-fashioned can cooler that pumps icy water over the milk cans stands a brand-new refrigerated bulk tank. The small vat pasteurizer was made in 1951, the year Jack was born. The water for it is heated by a medieval-looking wood-fired boiler, which came from a defunct local dairy. Naturally the Lazors use the lowest-temperature pasteurization method. Their post-and-beam barn was newly built by a young craftsman, and they moved an old wooden silo beside it. This is not entirely antiquarianism; old equipment is usually cheap.

Like other farm people, Jack and Anne Lazor are very straightforward as they speak. I found it easy to explain my criticism of the cream. Jack readily agreed, adding that the cream didn't whip well.

He was eager to correct the problem. From recent reading, I was sure that either agitation or heat caused the cream plug. We soon came up with a suspect. Jack and Anne were putting the cream through the old separator at 80 to 85 degrees Fahrenheit — much cooler than that and the machine would clog. But the melting point of butterfat is from about 90 to 96 degrees (a range because the fat is actually composed of various fats, or fatty acids). If the separator really was the culprit, there seemed to be no alternative but to replace it. It soon became clear that too many long hours of hard work had kept them from looking for a solution. Somewhat incredibly, no one from the state had ever pointed out the problem or suggested an answer.

Of course, Jack and Anne Lazor have ready access to both raw and pasteurized milk from the same herd, and on flavor their opinions are definite. At home they don't use pasteurized products. Jack says, "I like raw cream better. I've always thought our cream had a kind of shortbread quality to it." Anne emphasizes, "I like raw milk a lot better." She notices the cooked flavor created by pasteurization. "I don't know what it is about store milk, but I don't have any use for it at all." Jack finds a lack of sweetness in it.

I brought home both milk and cream in both raw and pasteurized forms to compare the tastes. The milk had been bottled during my visit, and back home the first difference I noticed was that by five o'clock the pasteurized milk had formed a distinct cream line, while the line in the raw milk remained blurred. (I took that as a further clue that heat might be causing the cream plug.) The Butterworks whole milk is about 5.5 percent fat in winter, almost two points higher than the average. The fat falls about half a point in summer.

I had drunk a certain amount of raw milk before, but I had never had the chance to compare raw and pasteurized milk and cream from the same farm. All the forms of Butterworks milk and cream were delicious. Naturally, the effect of pasteurization was more apparent in the cream. Pasteurized cream tastes stronger and simpler than raw cream, the flavor consisting mostly of hints of caramel and custard, while raw milk has subtly sweet fresh nuances that I think of as "flowery," though they aren't musky at all. I don't have a really apt description. However, pasteurized or raw, all good milk and cream are bland in the old sense of the word — suave — as well as in the sense of mild that has displaced it.

The following week Jack called with good news. The day before he had found that with steady attention he could run the milk through the separator at as low as 70 degrees, and twenty-four hours later there was no sign of cream plug in the bottles. The cream had a new consistency and it whipped well. The only drawback to the new temperature was that it produced less cream. But Jack didn't care; he was happy to have a better product.

Alerted, the same day I went to a health-food store and bought two bottles of Butterworks cream from the new batch. I rapidly whipped some into a stable foam. In a blind tasting, I sampled plain whipped Butterworks cream and plain whipped ultrapasteurized cream: The Butterworks pasteurized cream tasted like raw cream by comparison. In the second bottle of cream, some buttery foam did rise over the next couple of days, but very little. A narrow skim line formed, but I'd come to realize there is no harm in it; it merely confirms that the cream is not homogenized. With a light shake it disappears. I later compared the two kinds of whipped cream sweetened and flavored with vanilla. The difference remained marked.

Building on this success, when the farm's income allows it, Jack and Anne plan to buy a slightly higher-tech, used "in-line" separator, so they can lower the temperature further. The milk will enter and leave through piping rather than being poured in by hand.

I hear rumors of a resurgence in the production of truly good cream, but it will surely always be rare. At the risk of being overly romantic, I will say that I believe the cream with the most beguiling character is that which has had the least done to it. It comes from colored cows grazing on deep permanent pasture during late spring (or whatever the local season may be) when wildflowers are at their peak; the cream is neither pasteurized nor homogenized; it is chilled immediately after milking; and it is consumed shortly after.

16

Vanilla: Bourbon,
Mexican, and Tahitian

When I discovered Tahitian vanilla in the 1980s, about the time it first made a small splash in the American food world, I quickly came to prefer it, although all the older references and most current ones disparage the vanilla grown on Tahiti. "Mexican vanilla is regarded as the best," says the ninth edition of the *Encyclopaedia Britannica* (1890) — with scarcely a mention of Tahitian. Henry N. Ridley in *Spices* (1912) wrote that "the pods are poor in vanillin and have too strong a scent of heliotrope, or piperonal. For this reason the Tahiti vanilla can hardly be used at all as a condiment." The best modern reference, *Spices* by J.W. Purseglove et al., continues to dismiss Tahitian beans, saying they are "occasionally cultivated, but yield an inferior product." And Leslie Land, in a thoughtful piece about vanilla in *The Journal of Gastronomy*, concluded that "sources both antique and modern are united in citing Mexican vanilla as the *ne plus ultra* of vanilladom, possessing the fullest, roundest, most exquisite flavor." She adds, "But can you get any? You cannot." In Vera Cruz, region of traditional Mexican vanilla production, the switch to more lucrative citrus, cattle, and oil drilling has radically reduced the quantity of Mexican vanilla, and at the same time the quality has dropped. But these pro-Mexican opinions, heightened by the elusiveness of Mexican vanilla beans, lurked in the back of my mind until I began to doubt my Tahitian tastes. Do

199

traditional Mexican vanilla and the similar, almost as highly regarded Bourbon (mostly Madagascan) vanilla have special qualities that recommend them above all others? And what of vanilla's perplexing descent to plainness — "plain vanilla" — after several centuries of being esteemed as alluring and exotic?

Without human intervention, the vanilla pod develops no great interest. When the pod is picked from the vine, it is partially ripe and has almost no scent. The aroma develops as a result of a complicated process of curing that lasts five to six months or more after harvest. Left to itself on the vine, a vanilla pod continues to ripen until it splays open to disperse its tiny seeds. Eventually the pod blackens and develops a small amount of vanilla scent, which dissipates.

The first European known certainly to have tasted vanilla was Cortés, who in 1520 was offered a cup of vanilla-flavored chocolate by the soon-to-be-murdered Aztec emperor, Montezuma II. This was reportedly the only royal drink, and it probably contained other ingredients as well, making it a beverage we wouldn't recognize. Chocolate itself was not a rare food in Central and South America, but vanilla, *tlilxochitl* (literally "black pod"), was precious. Even so, ten years earlier, the first vanilla beans may have been sent back to Spain from Cuba, along with other New World gleanings. Apparently, this vanilla was considered perfume, not flavoring, and Cuba cannot have been its source. Vanilla was grown and cured by the Totonac Indians, who lived in the area of Vera Cruz and were one of the peoples conquered by the Aztecs. The Totonacs sent the emperor vanilla beans as tribute — for perfume and to flavor his *chocolatl*.

Only after a long delay did vanilla begin to be valued in Europe for flavoring. Hugh Morgan, apothecary to Queen Elizabeth, is supposed to have been the first to make the suggestion. It was in the 1600s through Spain that the taste for vanilla spread, along with the Spanish name, *vainilla*, "little pod" or "sheath." Its use broadened gradually from royalty to prosperous classes throughout the Continent. A measure of vanilla's popularity in Britain in the first half of the nineteenth century (recounted by Waverley Root) was the compliment paid by an aristocratic father to his daughter: "Ah, you flavor everything, you are the vanilla of society." For three hundred years, Mexico remained the source of the world's vanilla.

The vanilla vine is an orchid. In Mexico, the wild blossoms are or were pollinated by a small bee of the genus *Melipona*, by hummingbirds, and, perhaps, by ants. Cuttings of the vine were taken to other parts of the world and grown successfully there, but they almost never bore fruit. Finally in 1836, a Belgian botanist produced vanilla pods by hand-pollinating the flowers, and he deduced that outside Mexico the natural pollinators were missing. A few years later on the French island of Réunion in the Indian Ocean, Edmond Albius, a former slave, invented an efficient method for hand-pollination on a large scale, and his method is in use today: in essence, a worker bends aside the intervening parts of the flower with a splinter of bamboo and presses together the male anther and the female stigma. On Réunion, this was called *le mariage de vanille*. A nimble worker can fertilize fifteen hundred and up to two thousand flowers in a day. By 1886, more vanilla was grown in the islands of the Indian and Pacific oceans than in Mexico.

Until the French Revolution, Réunion was the Ile Bourbon, after the royal family (then for a time it was the Ile Bonaparte). The Bourbon name endures to describe the vanilla with the second-highest reputation for quality after Mexican. Most of it is actually grown on the northeastern coast of Madagascar, with smaller amounts coming from relatively nearby Réunion and the Comoro Islands. The Seychelles used to be famous for producing vanilla, but there, along with other problems, vanilla has been overtaken by tourism.

Today, what vanilla is grown in Mexico is still tended by the Totonacs. As everywhere, pollination is still carried out by hand. The original jungle is largely destroyed, and the Indians work on plantations owned by others. A few years ago, Coca-Cola and McCormick & Company (the largest US vanilla importer as well as producer of vanilla extract) tried together without success to reestablish large-scale vanilla production in the traditional area.

In quantity, the two major kinds are Bourbon from Madagascar and Indonesian, often still called Java, though it is now grown on other islands — Bali, Sumatra, Sulawesi. In the past, most of the Indonesian beans were picked far too green and then cured rapidly and badly. They were often dry enough to snap in half. Now much Indonesian vanilla is top quality, and within a few years Indonesia, already the source of most US vanilla, is expected to displace Madagascar as the dominant producer. Vanilla of some quality is also produced on the South Pacific islands of Tonga and Fiji and elsewhere. Yet aesthetically, a case might be made that the major kinds of vanilla are Bourbon (perhaps together with Indonesian), Mexican, and Tahitian.

All the many geographical kinds are divided into only two species. Mexican and Bourbon vanilla is *Vanilla planifolia,* and the kind restricted almost entirely to one South Pacific island is *Vanilla tahitensis.* Tahiti's beans are fatter, thicker skinned, and strongly flowery in scent compared with the more traditional *planifolia* vanilla. There is a third species, *Vanilla pompona,* or vanillon, which is still more flowery and contains much less of the characteristic vanilla flavor. It was grown in the Caribbean islands of Martinique and Guadeloupe, but it has probably fallen out of cultivation. It was used in perfumery and as an adulterant of *planifolia* vanilla.

All the vanilla produced in the French territory of Tahiti used to be exported to France, which reexported some to other European countries. (West Germany, for one, now imports Tahitian beans directly.) Tahiti's production has rebounded from a low point in the 1970s. The United States, which imported none a decade ago, currently takes half the beans. This is entirely the work of the largest exporter of Tahitian vanilla, Tahitian Import/Export in Los Angeles, which came into being solely for the purpose of importing Tahitian vanilla. The United States already consumed over half the world's *planifolia* vanilla. France was and is the second-largest buyer of vanilla.

Since vanilla isn't native to Tahiti, it is curious that the island ended up with its own species. Vanilla was brought to Tahiti from

Manila in the Philippines in 1848, but it is impossible to trace the spread of vanilla cultivars from New World to Old and to colonies in the tropics. The Tahitian vanilla plant may have been produced intentionally by crossbreeding (in the Philippines, according to rumor), or it may be that in nature the lines between species and strains are blurred. Growers in Tahiti distinguish as a matter of course between three distinctly flavored subspecies, each with a Tahitian name. In curing, the three are mingled together, and no one outside Tahiti is conscious of the differences.

It is difficult to find words for the qualities that all vanillas have in common. There is sweetness, richness, and depth — or complexity. Hank Kaestner, director of spice procurement at McCormick, says that experts at his company distinguish many fine nuances, and they can tell by aroma where a bean comes from. By reputation, Madagascan vanilla is particularly smooth and rich; Réunion has more sweetness and spice; Mexican is finer, with a hint of sharpness or pungency; Tahitian is, of course, exceptionally perfumed. Many traits are not fixed. Additional ones are creamy, woody, tobacco-like, chocolate-like, and leatherlike. Whether the differences result more from culture and curing or more from nature is hard to say. And while certain traits appear to be typical of one country or another, beans from the same country have been known to fluctuate remarkably in aroma.

In the wild in Mexico, in the shade of the jungle canopy vanilla vines climb trees, rising up fifty feet or more. Under cultivation, to keep the vines within reach, they are looped over specially planted trees or training stakes seven or eight feet tall. Normally, only one of the pale, yellow green blossoms in a cluster opens at a time. It does that early in the morning and must be pollinated before it begins to fade in midafternoon. Each blossom produces a single bean. Flowering lasts two months, and the vines are visited daily until the desired number of flowers has been successfully pollinated, roughly 150 on an average plant. The pods hang in banana-like bunches; long, straight pods bring a higher price. They grow for eight to nine months before they are harvested. Ripening proceeds from the blossom end, yellow gradually rising up the fruit.

The most important influence on the flavor of the beans, besides whether they belong to the Tahitian or *planifolia* species, is curing and conditioning. Methods vary. Bourbon beans are first "killed" by dipping baskets of them briefly into near-boiling water. This starts the reactions that produce the cure. In Mexico, the beans are first placed in sheds for several days to shrivel. Next, although ovens have sometimes been used, in the oldest method for both Bourbon and Mexican beans, they are laid out each day on wool blankets in the sun to bake until they are too hot to touch. At night, they are wrapped in their blankets and sealed up indoors to "sweat." This routine may continue for several weeks. The beans darken and shrivel, becoming flexible. Eventually, good beans turn chocolate brown to black. For two to three months more they are dried in the shade, and then they are tied in tight bundles and packed away for conditioning.

Sunning, sweating, and conditioning produce an intricate transformation. Certain complex substances break down into a much larger number of simpler ones. First, glucose and the dominant flavoring of vanillin are formed. Then, some of the vanillin is broken down into numerous other aromatic substances; more compounds are broken down in parallel fashion. And further changes occur through oxidation. Over 250 flavor components have been identified (not an unusual number in foods). The flavor compounds occur both in the walls of the bean and in the sticky seed-bearing gel inside. Vanillin is the main flavor substance (there is much less vanillin in Tahitian beans), but by itself, vanillin is one-dimensional. If it weren't, we would all probably use inexpensive artificial extract. Most of the volatile substances are insignificant individually, but in the aggregate they are essential to natural vanilla flavor.

Crystals of vanillin sometimes form on the outside of the beans, occasionally whitening them entirely. Any well-cured beans with good moisture content will form this *givre*, or "frost," if half a dozen or more are sealed in a jar. *Givre* indicates high quality, but when the beans are exposed to air, the *givre* sublimes — the chemist's apt verb for a solid changing directly to vapor. Those who buy only a few mediocre whole beans to use at home almost never see it, and *givre* does not form on Tahitian beans at all.

Planifolia vanilla pods are picked when they are mature but before they begin to turn yellow, because soon after that the capsule cracks up its length, greatly reducing its value. Tahitian vanilla may be picked more yellow because the pods do not open as quickly. But with either kind, the more ripe the pod, the larger the quantity of flavor precursors it contains — making a more flavorful bean after curing. The curer is usually a middleman who buys beans from the growers. If he buys beans that have almost begun to split, he will end up with a higher grade of cured beans. Splits don't matter much to the makers of vanilla extract, but they are unacceptable as whole beans for use in kitchens. About 95 percent of Tahitian beans go for the latter, so growers are wary of risking splits. The percentages are reversed in the trade in *planifolia* beans; almost all are destined for extract.

Bourbon beans are graded as firsts, seconds, thirds, and fourths. Firsts are oily looking, supple, brown-black, and they have strong aroma; the lower grades are progressively drier and weaker in scent. In Mexico, the classifications are similar. Tahitian vanilla beans for the United States are divided into three numerical grades. No matter the grade, most vanilla dealers evaluate the beans by appearance and aroma. They massage the bundle of a hundred or so beans in their hands to warm it and then they smell. By weight, vanilla is the second most expensive spice after saffron; white-husked cardamom is third.

The problem of "plain vanilla" must arise from vanilla's ubiquity as a flavor. And, of course, all but a tiny portion of the world's vanilla flavoring is avowedly artificial, solely or mostly vanillin, which is a by-product of liquid waste from softwood pulp used in paper manufacture.

Artificial vanilla is an ordinary flavor. Its omnipresence has certainly obscured exotic, complex natural vanilla, which is still an ingredient in expensive perfumes. Real vanilla shouldn't flavor everything.

The primary quality that vanilla contributes is sweetness, though that subtle sweetness is usually overwhelmed when a cook adds sugar. Vanilla's innate sweetness is quite clear in a cup of unsugared black coffee specially prepared with either Tahitian or Bourbon vanilla. (Allow one inch of vanilla bean per cup, and grind the vanilla with the coffee beans.) This vanilla coffee tastes a little too much like one of the commercial flavored coffees, but that's not the point of the exercise.

Three wonderful companions to vanilla in desserts are coffee, caramel, and chocolate. Their flavors play to vanilla's strengths, and chocolate almost requires it. Another flatterer is rum — golden and dark rum having flavor similar to caramel; still another is coconut. Vanilla superbly heightens the flavor of fresh fruit, especially tropical fruit. Vanilla's intricacy shows clearly in plain custard; ice cream is too cold for that. (The favorite recipe of one of the partners in Tahitian Import/Export is: split a papaya in half, remove the seeds, and put a pat of butter in each half. Cut a Tahitian vanilla bean lengthwise, cut it again into half-inch pieces, and put them into the papaya halves. Sprinkle with sugar and place the papaya in a 350 degree oven to warm and infuse for ten minutes. Remove the pieces of bean and top with Bourbon-vanilla ice cream.) I understand the role vanilla may play with certain seafood, and I can imagine that vanilla might work with such meats as rabbit, a combination some cooks have proposed. But I haven't explored those possibilities.

A simple use for whole beans is to make vanilla sugar. Bury a whole bean in a pint jar of granulated sugar or confectioners' sugar (if the bean is quite moist, it may cause some caking) and wait two weeks before using the sugar; replenish the jar periodically until the bean is spent. Or pulverize a bean with sugar in a food processor (one bean to two cups of granulated sugar or mixed granulated and confectioners') and strain the sugar through a fine strainer. An easy variation is to place a bean in a jar of honey. When beans are employed directly, they are usually steeped in the liquid called for in a preparation (the intact bean doesn't fleck the dish with seeds), or they are halved lengthwise and the seeds and gel scraped out and incorporated.

Vanilla beans should be stored in a tightly sealed glass jar so that they retain as much as possible of their moisture and volatile essence. Unless I have enough beans to nearly fill a jar, I put them first in a small plastic bag and then into the jar. They undergo further conditioning in the jar and keep indefinitely, until they dry out.

Extract, unlike whole beans, is readily available and effortless to use. Extract is made by circulating and recirculating a mix of alcohol and water through chopped beans in a sealed stainless-steel vat. That is generally done at 70 degrees Fahrenheit or less to preserve as many of the minor flavor notes as possible.

Just as vanilla beans are conditioned, vanilla extract, too, is usually aged, for three to six months. The aging normally occurs during the bottles' slow progress through retail channels, though some makers hold it for a time at the factory. The chemical transformations are like those in maturing wine, and the flavor becomes fuller and softer. Sugar is said to quicken aging. Brown bottles protect the contents from light, and the extract should be kept cool. Unopened bottles at McCormick have continued to improve for twenty-five years; they are said to be much better than ones that are only five years old.

The vanilla extract manufactured and sold in Mexico is generally fortified with coumarin, a dangerously toxic natural flavoring obtained from the tonka bean. There is supposed to be a little pure Mexican extract made from time to time, but don't buy extract in Mexico, especially at a bargain price, unless you are certain of the purity of the contents. Until 1954, when coumarin was banned in the United States, its very sweet flavor was widely employed in artificial and blended vanilla extracts. Chat Nielsen, president of Nielsen-Massey Vanillas, second-largest American extractor, says, "People used to love that flavor." At the time coumarin was made illegal, he weaned his customers batch by batch, reducing the coumarin by 10 percent each time.

Now, Nielsen-Massey makes only pure vanilla extract from Bourbon and, on occasion, Mexican beans. Chat Nielsen thinks the Mexican are "just slightly" superior. "I don't really care for Tahitian." I asked him if he believes a whole bean is ever superior to extract. "Basically, I don't feel it is." He considers extract to be more consistent and reliable and easier to disperse in, say, a cake batter.

On the other hand, Hank Kaestner of McCormick says, "The bean is superior in all cases. The flavor is very much better than extract." He thinks the limitation is that Americans may be offended at finding pieces of vanilla bean in their food. Extractors precipitate out sediment before bottling so that it won't form later and trouble the consumer. The sensory experts at McCormick aren't sure exactly what sediment contributes to flavor, but they know it contributes something, and that something is lost when sediment is eliminated.

I've accumulated bottles of extract from six or eight different producers, though not the less-expensive brands, which are simply made from fewer and sometimes inferior beans. I haven't evaluated my collection with formal blind tastings, but certainly Nielsen-Massey (sold by Williams-Sonoma) is high quality, reminiscent of pints of expensive vanilla ice cream, the use to which most of the brand is put. And McCormick's *planifolia* (mostly Bourbon) extract is good, a trifle different from Nielsen-Massey's. The others are fine but either less intense or with hints of off-flavors. And Tahitian Import/Export contracts to have a Tahitian extract produced. Of all the bottles, the most unusual is a steam-distilled essence from the old perfume center of Grasse in Provence; it has no alcohol at all, but heat appears to have altered its flavor and it belongs in a lesser category.

After handling beans and comparing extracts, I'm convinced that the whole bean is the most complete, superior form of vanilla. Extract can't possibly contain all the fugitive flavors of the bean — or else they have been transformed and diminished. And extract sometimes adds an undesirable alcohol taste to food. Serious professional chefs prefer the whole bean, which is also a sensual pleasure to handle.

The best beans are particularly supple from moisture. During curing and conditioning, moisture declines from 80 percent to 28 or 29 percent in a top-quality Bourbon or Mexican bean and about 35 percent in a Tahitian bean. These percentages may be ideal, but they are compromises. A more moist bean will continue to develop, change, and concentrate, but it can mold. (The Tahitian tolerates a little more moisture without molding.) If the bean is too dry, it loses volatile flavors faster than it gains them. A dry bean is usually a poor one.

Unfortunately, virtually all the whole beans for the US retail trade are simply dry beans diverted from the supply intended for extractors. Because extractors don't want to pay for water, they prefer beans that have dropped to 25 percent moisture, and 20 percent is not uncommon. These Bourbon beans are classified as thirds and fourths. The whole Tahitian beans sold here are impressive partly because they are so plump, fleshy, and soft compared with the usual dry kind. Yet Bourbon beans do exist that are almost as moist and fat as the Tahitian. These are Bourbon firsts and seconds, and virtually all go to Europe. However, there is at least one American importer of firsts, Tahitian Import/Export.

The world of American vanilla importers is small, no more than about a dozen people who know one another and occasionally sell back and forth to help each another out, though they are in competition. One of this group, a knowledgeable man who speaks with interest and in depth about vanilla, warned me against having any romantic ideas about his career: "After a while, it's just work. You're not looking forward to going out to some exotic jungle to buy vanilla beans, because you're really going to sit down with Chinese middlemen in a stinky little godown somewhere. You're getting drunk with these guys — ." But another importer strongly dissents. He has traveled to producing areas more than fifty times, and he can't wait to go again.

When I began to write about vanilla, I strongly preferred the Tahitian. The flavor of Bourbon beans seemed to me too easily lost, even in custard — and especially when mixed with another flavor such as coffee. Floral Tahitian vanilla seemed to point itself out. But

Hank Kaestner takes a different view. "It's as if someone spilled perfume in the ice cream." Currently, I have in the house an inordinate
number of Tahitian beans, as well as Bourbon firsts from Madagascar, outstanding Balinese beans, dryish unnamed *planifolia* beans
(presumably thirds or fourths), *planifolia* beans from French Poly-
nesia, and even genuine top-quality Mexican beans — not impossible to find after all. They are moist and faintly peppery, hard not
to appreciate having heard so much about them. Any excellent bean,
Bourbon or Tahitian, is intoxicating to hold in your hand. In my
informal tastings and smellings, most people have preferred Tahitian
over more familiar Bourbon vanilla. (With ice creams served side by
side, guests couldn't detect the Bourbon vanilla flavor after they had
tasted the Tahitian ice cream. Another time, diners loved the new
flavor but couldn't put a name to it, not imagining the possibility of
more than one vanilla.) And I do, still, generally prefer the Tahitian,
but I am glad to find uses for both. To smell the beans in the kitchen
is to luxuriate for a moment in a small, happy, personal knowledge
of the tropics.

17

English Walnuts

The edible kernel of the English walnut, the nutmeat, is actually the two seed leaves of the walnut seed, like the two halves of a bean or pea, although in the walnut these leaves don't actually emerge when the seed sprouts. The flavor of the kernel comes from its two parts: the skin and the blond meat underneath.

The golden to dark brown papery skin is both bitter and astringent, providing a good part of walnut flavor. The bitterness and astringency come from tannin, which defends the oils of the nut against turning rancid (oxidizing). The amount of tannin is reflected partly in the color of the skin. Darker skins are not necessarily, as you might think, more tannic; often lighter skins are. Some walnut varieties produce lighter or darker skins than others, and the skins are lighter if the nuts are harvested slightly less mature. After the harvest, the skin darkens somewhat with age. Yet the walnut industry here and abroad believes the skin should always be light because consumers judge quality by appearance — in walnuts by light color.

Light or dark, the taste of the skin is attractive coupled with the rest of the mild nut flavor. Without the skin, walnut flavor is nearly lost in some combinations. But the skins can give too much flavor. I once baked a cake using a high proportion of reasonably fresh walnuts to flour, and it tasted as if it had been made from stale whole-wheat flour, which is also somewhat bitter (from rancidity, not tannin).

Nearly all American walnuts and a quarter of the world's walnuts are now grown in California (France used to be the largest producer), primarily in the four-hundred-mile-long Central Valley. The dry climate there defeats walnut blight, which otherwise attacks leaves and developing nutlets. In California, walnut trees generally leaf in mid-March after the rainy season is over, yet they are irrigated during the rainless summer.

Walnuts are harvested when the green outer husk begins to crack, the thin divider separating the halves of the kernel is no longer leathery but brittle, and the kernel itself is still quite moist. In California, the nuts used to be knocked down by bamboo poles and dried in the sun. Now in large plantings there, the nuts are brought to the ground by a mobile trunk shaker; machines sweep them into windrows; other machines gather them up; and then they are mechanically hulled, washed, and dried to 8 percent moisture. Without drying, walnuts don't store long before turning rancid. The nuts to be sold in the shell are bleached — the matter of color again. Said Robert T. Morris, writer of a 1921 book on nut culture, "The general market in our country seems to call for bleached blondes a little off in character." But most shells don't have to be bleached because most nuts are sold as pieces.

Before they are dried, the freshly picked crisp, green walnuts are a quarter or more water. Abroad, these fresh nuts are picked about a dozen days before their natural fall, and they are enjoyed during a short season from the end of September through October. They must be peeled, or the bitter skin gives a somewhat painful reaction in the mouth. Peeling is a slow after-dinner occupation.

In similar fashion, the skin of regular dried walnuts is removed for some preparations. The flavor is more delicate, and in a light-colored preparation, if the skins aren't removed, there may be discoloration. Some batches of nuts (perhaps fresher ones) give up their skins more easily than others. It is surprisingly easy to remove most of the skins by baking the nuts for ten minutes at 325 degrees Fahrenheit and then rubbing them vigorously in a kitchen towel. The aim is to heat the nuts sufficiently to loosen the skins but not enough to produce an emphatic toasted flavor. The skins can be completely removed without any toasting — at a great cost of tedium — by pouring a generous amount of boiling water over the meats and letting them soak for two minutes before beginning to peel them one by one. This untoasted skinned nut is considerably more subtle in taste.

A dried walnut is more than half oil. But the unsaturated oils in both walnuts and hazelnuts are prone to rancidity, a problem that is often apparent in the pressed nut oils used mostly for salads. And it seems that most of the imported nut oils are not as good as the powerful, slightly cloudy oils pressed in the few remaining old mills of France. It is said that at one time, half the oil used in France was walnut oil. There cooks often dilute nut oils with olive oil or another oil on the grounds that they are too strong by themselves, but then most French cooks like fairly mild olive oil, too. Nuts and their oils should be kept cold and away from light and air by storing them in jars in the refrigerator; better yet, nuts can go in the freezer.

Besides the familiar multitude of dessert uses, walnuts are increasingly used in salads, where they provide a flavorful balance to fruits and strong greens like watercress. The nuts go especially well with dill, garlic, and parsley. Walnuts reduced to a paste bind and thicken certain sauces, usually garlic sauces such as pesto (when walnuts are used instead of pine nuts) or the *aillade* of Toulouse, which is an olive oil–walnut emulsion like a yolkless version of *aïoli*, the Provençal garlic mayonnaise. And there are walnut sauces specifically for fish. Walnuts also suit Roquefort and certain other cheeses, as well as port and sherry, combinations that can be exploited in cooking.

Americans call the usual walnuts "English walnuts," because once they were imported by way of the mother country, although they weren't grown there. The name English distinguished these walnuts from the edible native black walnut, the California black walnut, and the butternut. Ironically, although walnut trees grow well enough in Britain, in the damp, cool climate they don't reliably bear nuts. Young leaves and flowers are killed by the lightest spring frost, eliminating the year's crop. And the dampness abets walnut blight. Britain currently produces as few walnuts as it has in centuries; almost all of Britain's walnuts are imported.

Overall, however, the English walnut is the most widely grown nut in the world, since the tree tolerates both winter temperatures well below freezing and subtropical summers. In Persia, walnuts have been cultivated for at least several thousand years. From there, the trees spread to the Levant and then to Greece, where the nut was called the Persicon (or Persian walnut, which is today the common name among professionals and the English). In Rome, the walnut was known as *jovis glans*, "the acorn of Jove." (In botanical Latin the name became *Juglans regia*; the redundant addition means "royal.") The walnut was probably first planted in England during the eleventh century, when our word *walnut* appeared. It means "foreign nut," in reference to France and Italy.

The first walnuts planted in California were probably brought from Chile around 1770 by Franciscan fathers. These Mission, or Los Angeles, trees were propagated from seed, and they bore a fair crop around Los Angeles, but farther north the flowers were often killed by late frosts. French walnuts were better suited to the cooler climate. And in the late nineteenth century, all the important French varieties were brought to California both as seed and as grafting wood. The French were the most intent selectors of varieties and the first to reproduce them in a significant way by grafting, so that above the graft every tree in a stand was identical. In California, many seeds of the French stock and its progeny were planted on the chance that some seedling might prove to be a valuable variety. A number of new varieties were selected, and they gradually replaced the old Mission. Only in the 1940s at the University of California at Davis was a breeding program of intentional crosses begun.

Nuts of different varieties vary in size, shape, flavor, astringency, tenderness, shell thickness, tightness of the seal between the two halves (tightly sealed nuts keep longer), and proportion of meat to shell (small meats reduce the yield, but too big and the kernel can't be pried loose). Among old French varieties, the Barthère is up to two and a half inches long though only half as wide; the Gant, or Bijou, is about two inches across and was once used to hold a pair of ladies' gloves or fashioned into a jewel case; and the Mesange has the thinnest shell of any variety, so thin that in France it is pecked through by the small lark called a *mésange*.

Three very old French varieties, Franquette, Mayette, and Parisienne, set the standard for eating quality in California well into the twentieth century. Today, Franquette is declining in California, though the variety still makes up a tenth or more of the crop. And in France, Franquette is by far the most common variety in new plantings. The area around Grenoble is especially known for walnuts and has its own controlled place-name. The *noix de Grenoble* must be either a Franquette (as nearly all are), a Parisienne, or a Mayette. Unfortunately, the last is scarcely planted in spite of its eating quality, because it is susceptible to walnut blight. All three varieties come from the same bank of the Isère in or near the town of Vinay, not far from Grenoble.

In California, Franquette has largely been displaced by Hartley, now the most common California walnut. The first Hartley, from a seed planted in 1892, was grown by Mr. and Mrs. John Hartley on their property near the town of Napa. The nuts are said to have won a blue ribbon in 1915 at the International Exposition in San Francisco. But the Napa Valley wasn't a walnut district, and the variety languished until 1930 when two local farm advisers brought it to San Joaquin County in the Central Valley; from there, it quickly spread. Now almost all walnuts exported or sold here in the shell are Hartleys. On the world market they compete with European Franquettes.

In the varieties that become popular with growers, productivity, including disease resistance, takes precedence over other virtues. One variety that achieved a small, local fame before it went into eclipse is Poe. I learned of Poe in the 1980s when I visited the ranch of Chris and Jan Twohy near Lakeport in northern California. Lake County is not a major walnut-producing area, and the Twohys' main product is goat's milk cheese, including two exceptional aged cheeses. But they also tend an old stand of Poe walnut trees. Poes are much less astringent than most walnuts, so the underlying nut flavor shows clearly — to me, partly butterscotch. The shell is tightly sealed. The Poe's shortcomings are a slightly thick shell and low and inconsistent yields.

The Twohys' ranch is certified organic. Since Lake County is higher and cooler than the Central Valley, walnut trees aren't bothered by many insects. They have to be irrigated at most twice a year, and the relatively dry conditions of the climate and infrequent irrigation favor organic methods. The conditions probably also favor higher-quality nuts. In the fertile big valley, walnut growers feel they are losing money if they don't get two tons an acre, but with the lower land prices in Lake County, growers are content with half a ton per acre.

By asking old-timers, Chris Twohy learned that the Poe variety came originally from a farm only six miles away. The variety was selected by Oscar Poe around 1900 from a number of seedlings he had planted. His descendants still remember Great-Uncle Oscar, who was a kind of local Johnny Appleseed of walnuts. The Poe walnut was never planted much outside its home territory, but people in Lake County still think it is the best-tasting walnut.

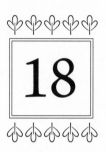

18

A Cup of Coffee

A powerful balm of freshly roasted and ground coffee permeates the tasting room in any of the tiny number of coffee-roasting companies that are truly serious about flavor. And a parallel intensity, a near-obsession, informs the coffee conversation of these companies' buyers and roasters (the people who do the actual roasting): Dave Olsen and Kevin Knox of Starbucks in Seattle, George Howell of the Coffee Connection in Boston, Tim McCormack of Caravali Coffees in Seattle, Dan Cox of Green Mountain Coffee Roasters in Vermont, Bob Rivkin of Schapira's Coffee in upstate New York, and more. To ask one of them a question is often to be besieged by words. They are eager to explain coffee flavor, coffee chemistry, roasting, details of harvesting and processing, consumer psychology, coffee economics, Third World politics, and geography (a wall-sized map of the world is de rigueur in tasting rooms). There is so much to tell. But most of all, these professionals are obsessed with quality. Specialty roasters deal in the fraction of the world's coffees that are top in quality and price, which they sell largely in their own stores. They now sell about 10 percent of American coffee.

The buyers and roasters of specialty coffee taste — "cup," as they say — an extraordinary amount of coffee. They sample each lot they consider buying. First, they look at the green beans, which are small, heavy, pale green versions of roasted beans and seem like jade. The tasters look for even-sized beans, medium to large for their type, and they note the exact shape and color, the amount of thin silverskin clinging to each bean, and the number of broken and discolored beans. They check for a clean grass or herb aroma. Then they roast a few ounces in a sample roaster. A number of samples are tasted at once, with the cups lined up in a considered order. Usually, the scraps of paper identifying them are turned face down. Into each cup go seven and a quarter grams of ground beans (the weight of a nickel plus a dime) and 150 milliliters of near-boiling water (about 5 ounces). Normally, some whole roasted beans from each sample (and sometimes ground coffee or green beans) are placed behind the liquid brewed from them to show the color of the roast and the nature of the beans. And several cups of the same coffee are lined up side by side, because slight flavor differences are produced by the particular beans that end up in a cup (one bad bean can spoil a sample). Or there may be side-by-side cups made from beans roasted to different shades. When the grounds have infused for about three minutes, the first taster breaks the airy, swollen crust of grounds with his round-bowled spoon to release a burst of aroma (which he aggressively inhales) and to force most of the grounds to the bottom of the cup. Tasters suck loudly from their spoons in a near hiss, taking in the liquid with plenty of air. They thoughtfully massage the drink with their tongues and move it about their mouths. Then they eject it into a spittoon. Swallowing would take its toll on the stomach, and the caffeine could build to a high pitch.

Inside the tasting room and wherever professional coffee people talk among themselves, the main characteristic that they talk about is *acidity*, which is also the most cautiously mentioned, or carefully unmentioned, topic when they talk with customers. "I always tell my staff never to use the word 'acidity,'" says the owner of one company. The public is afraid of acidity, the taste and the consequences to the stomach. Yet acidity is as necessary to the flavor of coffee as it is to the excitement of other drinks. And coffee is less acidic than beer, wine, or apple juice. For fear of being misunderstood, professionals speak not of acidity but of its effect on the palate. They refer to brightness, liveliness, snap, sharpness, sparkle, zest. A model of excellent, very brisk, high-acid coffee is Kenyan. Although you might assume that the acidity in roast coffee tastes blankly tart, specific acids contribute specific flavors, including burnt, caramel, butter, cream, chocolate, nut, and, somewhat generically, fruit. (Putting a name to a flavor clarifies it for the unaccustomed taster, but the adjectives are often inadequate. Two coffees described by the same words may be quite distinct.) In the course of roasting, the proportion of acids tends to diminish to more pleasing levels, and the chemical nature of the acids is altered. Lighter roasts retain more acidity, sometimes to a fault; the acids in darker roasts have begun to be driven off. The oily-dark roasts that Americans normally use for espresso are the least acidic of all.

Even if you don't drink coffee to excess, too much favorably acidic coffee is wearing and requires moderation in consumption. To taste three roasts of coffee from darker to slightly lighter reveals an increasing and displeasing acidity in the lighter roasts. After cupping a group of especially good acidic coffees, the taste of a dark roast can be a relief. How does one explain the paradox that acidity that shows badly in tastings is actually good? The answer lies in the inherent disadvantage of comparative tastings of food or drink. The examples compete against one another rather than interact with the foods that normally accompany them. Coffee doesn't go with coffee but with breakfast, say, or cake, where its mild acidity appears as an advantage, or it follows a meal — an accompaniment, so to speak, to repletion.

Coffee flavor, like other flavors, is built on the four basic tastes (sweet, sour, bitter, and salty) plus all-important aroma, which is carried on coffee's body of suspended fine particles and accentuated by tiny surface droplets of oil, enough of which contribute a creamy or buttery sensation. These components are played upon by a measure of dryness, or astringency. There is such a thing as too little body, but it's not exactly true that the more the better. Certainly, you wouldn't want to miss a flavorful coffee simply because its body was light. The balance and intensity of all the elements depend on the particular bean.

Balance is partly interaction. The trio of bitterness, sourness, and astringency reinforce one another, and they are easily mistaken for one another by unpracticed tasters. George Howell of the Coffee Connection observes of his customers, "They never say 'sour,' they always say 'bitter.'" Some bitterness is needed in coffee, but bitterness is virtually ignored among professionals (except growers, who see it entirely as a defect, since powerful bitterness can come from mistakes in processing the green coffee). Ted Lingle, a California roaster, intensively analyzed coffee flavor for *The Coffee Cuppers' Handbook*. He employed a neatly graphic triangle to show relationships among acidity, sweetness, and salt, but he made no place for bitterness. I grant that bitterness is a simple taste with little interest on its own and that we have an innate aversion to it, but we can acquire a taste for it as an enjoyable counterpoint. Certainly bitterness is admired in traditionally cured olives, tonic (quinine) water, grapefruit, certain red wines, beer, chocolate, and coffee. Not surprisingly, coffee drinkers like bitter tastes more than noncoffee drinkers do.

Coffee also contains a distinct mineral saltiness once you are attuned to it. Salt sharpens acidity, and a small amount of it increases sweetness. Beyond that, salt and sweetness mask each other. Coffee's natural sweetness is often elusive, but it is gratifying when present. Sweetness delays the sensations of bitterness and astringency and makes them more palatable, and it diminishes the impression of acidity, as acidity diminishes the impression of sweetness.

Aftertaste is an important part of the taste of coffee. Often, it is reminiscent in an unexpected and pleasant way of the smell of fresh tobacco smoke. One also finds traces of wood smoke, caramel, chocolate, sometimes resin or spice. As most kinds of coffee cool, their flavor changes until the cold coffee has little to offer. When the more volatile, pleasant aromas disappear, they may unmask hidden shortcomings. Frequently, tasters return to a cold cup, partly in hope of finding one of those few outstanding coffees that retains satisfying flavors when cold.

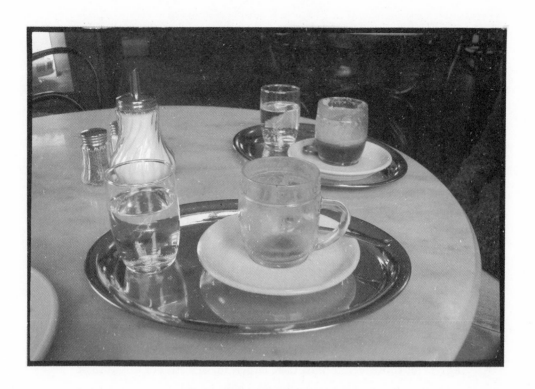

Viennese-style coffee at Café Sabarsky.
New York City, 2004.

A Cup of Coffee

The choice of coffee beans and roasting style (essentially, the color of the roasted beans) is at the heart of a roasting company. I've asked the buyers at several companies whose taste determines these choices, and each has answered: "It's my taste." As a rule, buyers start out as roasters, and the owners of some small businesses hold both jobs. The bigger specialty companies can afford to send their buyers to visit farms in the producing countries to learn more about coffee, to encourage quality production, and to discover outstanding growers. But almost no roasting company, even a mass-market one, imports coffee directly. Importing is the risky, specialized pursuit of brokers, who operate on the narrow margin of about a nickel a pound. Brokers, too, cup a lot of coffee.

When they cup, buyers decide whether to purchase a particular coffee and, if so, whether to blend it or sell it straight. The coffees they are most excited about have enough character and balance that the roasters prefer not to submerge their distinctions in a blend. On the other hand, canned supermarket coffees are always blends, and buyers for those blends must taste largely for defects. For this kind of cupping, the samples are roasted very light in order to show defects more readily. But the buyers for serious roasters look primarily for strengths, for unusually fine qualities. And most of the roasters I've visited taste coffee roasted to the same color as the coffee they sell, so it offers a full coffee taste. Even after years in the business, they take enormous pleasure in tasting.

All this tasting goes on because the flavor of any lot of beans is highly unpredictable. Myriad good and bad influences affect the beans during cultivation, processing, roasting, and even storage and shipping. Sudden, unexpected descents or ascents from previous standards occur, and no coffee is wholly consistent. Even from the same plot of earth, coffee is variable from year to year because of weather. But inconsistency also can come from poorly executed methods of cultivation, processing, or both, not so much from negligence on the part of growers as from ignorance. Many isolated growers have few technical resources and little opportunity to understand the connection between what they do and quality in the cup. Economic policies of Third World governments may reduce the incentive to produce a quality crop. A few famous old colonial coffee estates are completely government run, producing what is widely recognized as disappointing coffee.

Soil, climate, and other ingredients of *terroir* give the coffee from each growing region of the world a more or less characteristic taste. On a more local and subtle level, each farm or estate offers a variation on the theme. These individual flavors are preserved when a large farm or estate processes and markets its own coffee or when a group of small neighboring farms uses a cooperative processing plant. While the coffees they offer are sold at wholesale under their own marks, they are often unnamed at retail because supplies are insufficient to support sustained demand. The low point of interest in the quality of the world coffee crop came during the 1960s and 1970s, when there were scarcely any of these "single-estate" coffees; now there are thousands, including perhaps a few dozen superb ones.

Fine aromatic coffees come only from the species *Coffea arabica*, and the best arabicas are grown only at high elevations where the climate is both cool and relatively dry. Generally, the higher the better, from four thousand up to about six thousand feet, although coffee must never encounter frost. Cool, partly dry conditions produce a harder bean with more coffee aroma and acidity. Bill McAlpin of Tarrazu, Costa Rica, who is undoubtedly the world's most perfectionist grower, puts it this way: "More of everything comes from a harder bean."

The coffee in supermarket cans is blended largely from the species *C. canephora*, commonly known as robusta for its vigorous growth. Robusta grows more quickly than arabica and at lower elevations, where there is more moisture and heat. The robusta beans are smaller and softer, with less acidity. They brew into less expensive, more bitter, gray, flat-tasting coffee that contains about twice as much caffeine as arabica coffee. The United States' coffee consumption has been declining since the 1960s, and during that time robusta has increasingly entered most blends. The taste of canned coffee today is dismal. The recent popularity in the US of a large mug of weak coffee must be a result of the sour, green taste of mass-market underroasting (more profit per pound) plus the bitterness and lack of aroma typical of robustas. Weak is the only way to tolerate that kind of coffee. The problem was exacerbated in 1975, when the quality of coffee worldwide plummeted after 40 percent of the international coffee crop was destroyed by a frost in Brazil, the largest producer. Quality has yet to recover fully.

(Interestingly, what cannot be found in North America is a top-quality robusta, favored by some serious Italian roasters for blending with arabicas in a proportion of perhaps 15 or 20 percent. In such proportions it lends body and bitterness, its oils contribute to a larger amount of *crema*, and it increases the caffeine jolt that Italians admire. The very best robustas are said to form almost a third category of coffee.)

The drug caffeine is not to be dismissed as part of the essential nature of coffee. Aside from its contribution of bitterness, the wakefulness and alertness caffeine brings led to coffee's original extraordinary success first in the Islamic and then in the Christian world. Beyond clarifying and focusing the mind, it was formerly seen as increasing intelligence and wit. The tales may be apocryphal, but Balzac has been credited with drinking more than fifty cups of coffee a day, and Voltaire more than forty. Voltaire is supposed to have dismissed coffee's dangers, saying, "I have been poisoning myself for more than eighty years and I am not dead yet." Cafés and coffeehouses have played an important role in intellectual life.

"Doctors have propounded various opinions on the healthful properties of coffee, and have not always been able to agree." Brillat-Savarin's comment on the healthfulness of coffee suffices today (he was typically preoccupied with health as well as gastronomy). Caffeine is still controversial, but the reasonable consumption of coffee has not been definitely linked to health problems.

Coffee robbed of its caffeine is not the same drink. Dan Cox of

Green Mountain Coffee Roasters says, "I think we have some very, very good decaffeinated coffees. Do they stack up against the regular ones? No." The typical judgment among small roasters is that the main thing you do when you decaffeinate coffee is damage it. But every coffee company sells decaffeinated coffee because some people have trouble tolerating caffeine. Better an adequate cup of decaf than no coffee at all.

Roasters, however, have much less tolerance for flavored coffees, a liking for which is sometimes mistaken for the height of worldly discernment. No roaster respects flavored coffees; some refuse to sell them. The beans sacrificed to flavoring are never the very best, and the flavorings themselves lack dimension. They don't begin to measure up to the intricacies of flavor captured in a liqueur, which is a more reasonable addition to coffee. They certainly detract from that most sublime thing: a superlative cup.

The coffee-growing regions of the world lie between the Tropic of Capricorn and the Tropic of Cancer. Coffee is grown in Africa, Asia, in the Americas, and on far-flung islands. Some coffee is grown on large estates, but most is raised on small family farms, sometimes in mere plots. Millions of people depend on coffee for survival. The work is labor-intensive, but it often goes on in landscapes of extraordinary natural beauty.

A coffee tree produces only between three-quarters and one pound of green beans each year. The tree is less a tree than a large shrub that can reach twenty-five feet or more. The plant draws enormous amounts of nutrients from the soil, which the farmer must fertilize well. Soil provides much of the regional character of each coffee, and a particularly good soil produces beans of exceptional aroma, sweetness, and acidity. Coffee trees must be somewhat shaded by taller trees, or they must be grown close together on hillsides so that they shade one another. A coffee tree bears fruit relatively quickly — five years from seed to first crop — and modern varieties yield strongly for fifteen years. Cool and dry conditions reduce the need for pesticides, and in some areas the expense precludes even the use of chemical fertilizers. A few coffees, some very good, are grown organically by choice and are certified as such.

The white, jasmine-scented coffee blossoms appear following the start of the rainy season. Where the rainy season's beginning and end are poorly defined, the trees bear blossoms, green fruit, and ripe red cherries all at once. The cherry has no real flesh but only a mucilaginous pulp between the skin and the pair of seeds in the center. Usually, each of these beans is flattened on one side by the pressure of the other, but especially at the end of a branch, one bean in the cherry may go unpollinated and fail to form, so that the fruit is filled by a single rounded peaberry. The plump peaberries on a tree will be more intensely flavored than the predominating flat beans.

Ideally, only fully ripe cherries are picked. Says the grower Bill McAlpin, "It's probably the single thing the farmer can do to get the best out of what he's got." But to catch all the beans at a state of complete ripeness requires several harvests. And many farmers can harvest just once because of costs or a shortage of labor.

After the harvest, the seeds must be separated from the fruit pulp that surrounds them. The oldest method is to dry the cherries in the sun for two or three weeks and then mill off the brittle husk, including the underlying shell-like layer, called parchment. At least some of the thin silverskin adhering to the bean is removed at the same time. Originally, millstones were used, a method that may persist in Yemen. Such dry-processing results in arabica coffee that has less acid and more body as well as earthier, fruitier flavors than those found in the more common washed arabica coffee.

Washed coffee is produced where water is plentiful. Rather than drying the fruit in the sun and then grinding off the husk, the processor uses a brief alcoholic fermentation of the sweet fruit to free the seed. The fermentation must take place within twenty-four hours of picking, and it lasts from one to three days. If it goes on too long, the beans take on a barnyardy taste called "fermented," which shows plainly in the roasted coffee. The fermentation is ended by thoroughly washing away the pulp with large amounts of fresh water. Then the green beans are dried. Machine drying is now sometimes employed in place of sun drying; it sharpens acidity and increases astringency. Or the two methods are mixed to balance qualities. These days in Central and South America, enormous mechanical driers are used. Theoretically, moisture falls to 11.5 percent, but if the beans are taken too far in the heat, they lose aroma and acidity and take on a glasslike brittleness. On the other hand, if too much moisture remains, they mold. Too often, fermentation and drying proceed with little attention paid to such basics as using clean water and controlling times and temperatures.

After the washed beans are dried, the parchment and loose silverskin are rubbed off; further polishing can cause damage from heat. The whole of processing is called milling. Bill McAlpin explains, "When you take the fruit from the plant, it's at its best — if you did everything right. You can't improve on it, but you can make it enormously worse. The milling facility can certainly ruin what nature did."

Wet-processed beans are more lively — acidic — than dry-processed ones, and they have a cleaner, more clearly focused taste, less muddied by traces of unwanted flavors. You can tell the two kinds apart by color: washed beans are more blue; dry-processed are more yellow. Some countries use both methods, but generally the different qualities produced by the two techniques are inextricably tied to the character of a country's coffee. Dry beans from either process are sorted for color, size, and defects, all of which affect flavor. Highly sophisticated machines are common, although in some countries beans are still sorted by hand. It is often suggested, notably for true Mocha from North Yemen, that a few defects add to the complexity of a coffee's taste. But George Howell, of the Coffee Connection, says, "It's absolute bull to say the character is augmented by defects." He is considered by some to be the American most knowledgeable about regional differences in flavor, as well as the most finicky buyer. As an experiment, he asked an employee to sort a sample of already well-sorted top Antigua beans into three piles according to visible defects. In the best pile there was not even a trace of silverskin clinging to the beans, meaning they had been picked perfectly ripe. Then the three categories of beans were separately roasted and brewed. By comparison to the lesser piles, the taste of the best beans "was like having your window cleaned." Five hundred pounds of coffee cherries produce about one hundred pounds of green beans, which are sorted down to seventy to eighty pounds in the standard preparation for the American market and down to fifty to sixty pounds for European preparation (now requested by some Americans). What isn't good enough for export is, somewhat sadly, consumed within the producing country, where the coffee drunk is generally inferior (or, as in Indonesia, coffee is ignored and the common beverage is tea). As a rule, growers don't drink or taste their own coffee, so they readily switch to inferior, less costly growing practices and processing methods. Lately, many have planted the higher-yielding new variety called Catimor, whose poor flavor comes from its part-robusta background. One or two Americans in the coffee business have actually given a sample roaster to individual growers so that they could roast and taste their own coffee and understand the link between their methods and the taste in the cup.

The countries that grow arabica coffee can be broken down by flavor into three large geographic groups: East Africa, Indonesia, and the Americas. But among all coffees, George Howell discerns five or six that are flavor prototypes for the others. Probably no other coffee specialist would quite agree with all his choices and some would strongly dissent. But his five coffees are useful points of reference for considering differences in coffee flavor. They are Ethiopian, as exemplified by Yergacheffe; Mocha Mattari from North Yemen; Kenyan; Sumatran; and, taken together, Costa Rican and Antiguan, from the Antigua region of Guatemala. (The last two George Howell might separate, making a total of six).

Only arabica coffee is cultivated in Ethiopia, which contains the center of origin of the species. In the southwest of the country near the borders with Kenya and Sudan, unharvested wild trees cover thousands of acres. It is almost certain that coffee was first prepared as a drink in Ethiopia, and there the trees were first cultivated, perhaps a thousand years ago. Today particularly good coffee comes from the Ethiopian regions of Harar and Sidamo. Within Sidamo is Yergacheffe, in a portion of the Rift Valley between Addis Ababa and Kenya. Yergacheffe, grown at about five thousand feet, is one of the handful of top coffees in the world. (A *cheffe* is a valley where, during the rainy season, marshes form and tall grasses grow; *yerga* is to settle down.) Only since about 1980 has Yergacheffe been sold separately from the rest of Sidamo coffee. Like most Ethiopian coffee, it is washed, which enhances its naturally generous acidity. The flavor stands out for cleanness, brightness, balance, complexity, and a unique aftertaste of lemon peel, rising to the nose. It is, by consensus, the most flowery of all coffees.

Across the Red Sea from Ethiopia is Yemen, producer of Mocha, the oldest coffee in trade and the most famous; for more than two centuries it was regarded as the best. The coffee is named for the port of Mocha, once the center of the Yemeni coffee trade. The name is often applied indiscriminately to other coffees. But in the mountains of North Yemen, although coffee has been partly replaced by more lucrative and less-demanding bushes of *qat*, whose hallucinogenic leaves are chewed by many Yemenis, a much-diminished crop of real Mocha is still grown.

The first scant written records of coffee's use come from Yemen, where Sufi orders used it by the mid-1400s, apparently to keep awake during nighttime rituals. (Even today in Yemen, a sort of atavistic tealike drink, *qishr*, is made from the husk of the coffee fruit.) The drink soon achieved popularity, and its consumption steadily spread through the Islamic world, taking about a century to reach Istanbul. But a convulsive dispute arose within Islam, motivated largely by a disapproving reaction to the social innovation of the coffeehouse, which partly usurped the roles of the mosque and home. The Arabic word for coffee, *qahwa*, parent of the Western words for coffee, predates the appearance of coffee and was originally a term for wine. The etymology indicates the ambiguities in the perception of the drink. Was coffee not an intoxicant and prohibited like wine? Of course, in time coffee was found legal under religious law.

Coffee reached Europe through Islam. The first café in Vienna was opened after the Turks besieged the city in 1683. The proprietor was Franz George Kolschitzky, who, after the Turks were routed, was one of the rare Europeans who knew the use of the green beans they left behind. In Paris, the first highly successful café was La Procope, established by the Italian Francesco Procopio in 1686 and still in business today as a restaurant. And in London the first coffeehouse, at least of a sort, was opened about 1652 by Pasqua Rosée, Greek servant of an English merchant who had learned to drink his coffee in Turkey.

A handful of unroasted Mocha Mattari beans (from the Yemeni province of Bany Matar, generally the most highly regarded Mocha) is a yellowish and oddly irregular collection of small sizes. The color of the roasted beans is more uneven than that of any other coffee. What would be defects in appearance and flavor in coffee from elsewhere are construed as virtues in Mocha. The flavor is the most unusual of any coffee. All Mocha beans are dry-processed, and their acidity is only a step below Yergacheffe's. Mocha flavor is typically described as fruity and spicy, and supposedly it sometimes tastes of chocolate. I've never found that, and roasters say it is rare. (Presumably, though, it explains the leap to the coffee-chocolate combination called mocha. Some Guatemalan and Costa Rican coffees are by contrast quite clearly chocolatey.) The curious, salient feature of Mocha, however, is its dominant taste of fermentation, as if the brief fermentation of wet processing had gone too far and been allowed to impregnate the bean.

In Mocha beans, the flavor isn't usually identified as fermentation or considered exactly a fault. Either it's admired or the reaction is like that of Bob Rivkin, buyer and roaster at Schapira's Coffee in Pine Plains, New York: "It's extremely muddled, busy, and confusing. It's just too wild." Since Mocha is dry-processed, the fermentation can only occur within the fruit while it is drying. Unfortunately, information on coffee growing inside North Yemen is scant. But I have read that in the steep mountain terrain where coffee is grown on terraces, many of which are held back by stone walls taller than the growing area is wide, moisture for growing coffee comes more from heavy nighttime mists than from rainfall. (Some irrigation is also essential, and a system of ancient underground aqueducts brings water from higher in the mountains.) Maybe the drying coffee beans aren't protected from the mists, which encourage the fermentation. Can today's Mocha be the same as the one that took all fashionable Europe by storm and that remained the most admired of coffees well into the nineteenth century, after coffee was being produced in many European colonies?

Kenya, like Yemen and Ethiopia, grows arabica, and the better coffee is grown at higher elevations. AA is the grade of largest beans, superior to AB from the same source. Kenyan coffee is washed, and it has, if anything, greater acidity than Ethiopian. The acids are balanced by medium to heavy body and by other concentrated flavors, making a rich coffee. Related character is found in Tanzanian and Zimbabwean coffee. But in Zimbabwe the government acts as selling agent for all coffee, and individual farms and estates are not marked. The top grade is simply 053. This undercutting of the urge to produce quality probably explains Zimbabwean coffee's reputation as a poor man's Kenyan, although some superior lots do come through. In Tanzania, much is made of peaberries, sold separately at a premium. But here, too, coffee is said to suffer from the role taken by government.

In the Western Hemisphere, both Guatemala and Costa Rica produce fine washed coffees that are heavy-bodied and contain high acidity, together with fruit and nut flavors. The two kinds of coffee are more distinct than the words imply. You might generalize that

Guatemalan suggests smoke and spice, and certainly it is less clean than Costa Rican coffee, because processing technology in Guatemala is less advanced. The highest-elevation Guatemalan coffees are classified "strictly hard bean," and the most admired region is Antigua. In another part of the country, the department with the wonderful name of Huehuetenango produces especially rewarding coffee.

In Costa Rica, the finest growing region is Tarrazu, named for the Tarrazu River. Some plantings appear so dangerously steep as to be impossible to tend and harvest. The Tarrazu estate of La Minita is owned by Bill McAlpin, and its coffee is the most carefully, even fanatically, cultivated and processed in the world. Whether it is also the best is, of course, a matter of taste. Sixty to seventy women return year after year to sort the beans by hand. Eighty percent are rejected, so the taste is the cleanest possible, utterly unmuddied by imperfect beans. Tim McCormack, buyer for Caravali Coffees, has visited the farm, and he was impressed by the smell at the La Minita mill: "It smelled like this wonderful tropical fruit" — the ripe coffee cherry — while most mills smell like "rotting fruit." For obvious reasons, La Minita is among the most expensive coffees.

The last of George Howell's five flavor prototypes is Sumatran, a relatively low-grown coffee that is the exception to the high-grown rule. It is dry-processed and has exceptionally full body and strong character. Because the quality of Javanese coffee has declined in recent years, Sumatran is perhaps the best representative of the Indonesian style; the Mandehling district has long had the top reputation. (I find that Javanese sometimes has a slight rubber taste, not especially enjoyable. But one purist-minded coffee buyer, Dave Olsen of Starbucks, finds instead black pepper and leather.)

And then there is the special category of *aged* Indonesian coffee, descended from the historical practice of aging beans in the holds of sailing ships. All green coffee grows old in time, drying out and losing acidity, turning tan and then brown. Year-old beans, the only ones available shortly before the new crop arrives, have lost at least an edge of flavor. But when very good coffee is stored under conditions of ideal humidity, after about two years it gains an admirable mellow, nutty richness.

Of other areas, coffee grown in Colombia is all arabica, but despite the propaganda on its behalf, it isn't regarded as particularly special in the coffee world. Formerly, all Colombian coffee was mixed and sold together. Now some regions are distinguished, and recently a few American roasters have located one or two that stand out. Supremos are the largest-sized beans, but the smaller Excelso can be equally good.

Hawaiian coffee, which nearly all comes from the Kona district, has so great an appeal because of its exotic association that it manages to be overpriced despite its unexciting quality. Of course, it's more expensive to produce coffee in Hawaii than it is in Third World countries, and as a crop in Hawaii it suffers competition from more profitable macadamia nuts. Unfortunately, Hawaiian coffee isn't grown high enough. Bob Rivkin sums up, "At its best, it's a perfectly good coffee, but you wouldn't accuse it of being complex."

Less good and more overpriced is the famous Jamaican Blue Mountain coffee. In its ideal manifestation, it is supposed to show exceptional balance between moderate acidity and body, but no one I've asked claims to have encountered this. Apparently, the problem is that today most of the coffee is not well grown. The best-known estate, Wallenford, is government run and neglected. Dan Cox of Green Mountain Coffee Roasters: "When you get there, it's almost depressing." However, a small quantity of Blue Mountain is supposed to be impeccably produced, and it is bought at an exceptional price by the Japanese, who in the late twentieth century took up the connoisseurship of coffee.

In Europe, as formerly in the United States, it is usually taken for granted that there is more to be gained from blending good coffee than from consuming a single variety alone. The coffees chosen for a blend should be processed with equal care (so as not to dirty the taste of a clean coffee), and their strengths should be complementary; the result should always be greater aromatic complexity. The oldest blend is Mocha with Javanese, a combination of the first two coffees in commerce. Nowadays, good Mocha and Javanese are scarce, and a more usual combination is high-acid Kenyan or Central American coffee plus mellow and full-bodied Sumatran or other Indonesian coffee. I had thought, when I began to write, that a description of regional types would logically conclude with a thorough presentation of blends. But there is so much to learn about the different straight coffees that I haven't advanced to much understanding of blends. And, although they are the basis of espresso and of some people's understanding of coffee, they may not be of primary importance.

To name certain coffees as outstanding is to risk rebuttal by many other people who advocate alternatives with equal passion. I don't mean to exclude any plausible coffee from anyone's consideration: a budding coffee enthusiast should sample coffees from New Guinea, Mexico, Colombia, Peru, the Indonesian islands of Sulawesi (Celebes), perhaps Brazil's better arabicas (mostly, Brazil grows a sea of inferior arabica), and arabicas from various African countries as they are available from a roaster. Even after discovering a preference, it would be boring to stick to it. None of the specialty buyers I've asked has settled on one coffee or even a region; they take home a succession of different top coffees.

An odd and somewhat incomprehensible disagreement exists among American coffee specialists over the simple, important point of how dark to roast coffee beans. Scarcely anyone allows that this is a matter of taste. From reading the professional coffee literature and from conversations with roasters and buyers, I've come to the conclusion that for each batch of beans from each coffee-growing spot in the world there is an ideal degree of roasting that brings out maximum flavor. Too light a roast doesn't develop all the aromatics and sugars and doesn't transform and reduce the acids. Too dark a roast drives off much of the aroma, destroys acid, and ultimately reduces the coffee to a barren bitterness. Clearly, harder and larger beans require more heat, and softer and smaller beans require less. Naturally, there are finer points. I put my early conclusions about this ideal point of roasting for each lot of beans to George Howell, and he responded, "What's ironic is that everybody in the business would agree with you, but none of them would agree what that point is."

A particular color of roast can be reached by different combinations of heat, time, and draft. "There is an art to it, and experience is what counts in roasting as in tasting," says Tim McCormack, who was a roaster for five years. Normally, good arabica beans are roasted from twelve to twenty minutes at between 420 and 500 degrees Fahrenheit. The silverskin loosens and is carried away with the exhaust; otherwise this chaff would add its papery taste to the brewed coffee. Along the way, acids change and diminish, and if all goes well a caramel sweetness develops. The goal is to roast quickly but evenly. Roasting too fast finishes the outside of the bean before the inside is done; roasting too slowly bakes the aromatics out of the bean without creating the desired chemical changes. By a roaster's standards, even twenty or thirty extra seconds can result in a slight overroast.

After eight or nine minutes, the beans pop and double in size, assuming a thirteen- to fourteen-minute roast. And at twelve or thirteen minutes the beans again pop loudly, as the cell structure breaks and oil begins to leak to the surface. This second pop divides the roasters: some stop short of it, some stop in the middle, and others go well past. Beans roasted just to the second crack release some oil over the next day and then slowly reabsorb it. If the roast is taken much beyond the second crack, enough oil is released that it remains as a high gloss on the beans. Whatever the desired point, as soon as it is reached, the beans are dropped into a cooling tray and cooled by air currents or quenched with a fine water mist. At this point, flavor is somewhat muted. Tim McCormack again: "They really tend to open overnight; it's kind of remarkable." Roasters who specialize in darker roasts consider the improvement more marked, and I suspect the change applies more to darker roasts.

Three traditional American roasts, short of the dark roasts, are distinguished by color: cinnamon roast, city roast, and full-city roast. Cinnamon describes the pale brown coffee, an absurd under-roasting, still found at one store in Manhattan. Maybe the reason is economic; lighter roasts lose less weight. "I can't believe people buy it twice, but apparently they do," says a respected small roaster in another part of town.

The meaning of cinnamon is fairly clear, but the meanings of city roast and full-city roast aren't. The standard old industry reference, William H. Ukers' *All About Coffee* from 1935, never clearly addresses roasting color in its eight hundred pages, as far as I can see, except in one color illustration (if the color is accurate). In a discussion of coffee customs in Italy, Ukers writes, "The full-city, or Italian, roast is preferred." But he doesn't mention the complication of the progressively darker roast as one moves south down the boot.

The notion that darker is more sophisticated is foolishness. Generally, the most affluent European countries (notably Germany, Switzerland, and those of Scandinavia) buy the best coffees, and they roast them relatively light. It is the poorer southern Europeans who drink the darkest coffee, including the southern Italians, who brought their tastes to the United States. In fact, the origins of the dark roasts lie partly in their ability to transform inferior beans. But such subterfuge has nothing to do with what is happening in Seattle today.

During the 1980s, Seattle became the coffee capital of the United States. Its extraordinary number of indoor espresso bars and outdoor carts is unlike anything anywhere else in the country — or for that matter in Italy. Within a four-block radius of Pine Street and Fifth Avenue in downtown Seattle, there are about thirty different places to buy espresso. Much of this coffee is made perfectly from exactly the right proportion of tamped grounds to pressurized hot water and with a thick layer of tan *crema* on top. (The *crema* is the foam that pours out naturally with the coffee, arising from the oils, not from anything added.) Always, the beans appear to be top quality, freshly roasted and freshly ground.

Why Seattle? ask incredulous people elsewhere. Seattleites point to the rainy weather, the large number of Scandinavians with their love for coffee, a total population small enough to be influenced by word of mouth, a certain open-mindedness, and the many people who have chosen to live in Seattle for its quality of life, which easily takes in well-made Washington State wines and a good cup of coffee. At least as important is that in the 1970s two serious roasting companies happened to start up business in Seattle. The one called Starbucks became by far the largest specialty roaster in America; it spent fifteen years educating people about good coffee. By the early 1990s, Starbucks had forty-five stores around Seattle and ninety altogether, including twenty-two in Chicago. Each store contains an espresso bar. Starbucks' roast is distinctly dark. Even the basic roast is darker than most Europeans use for espresso, and the dark roasts are darker still.

The dark Seattle style originated in the late 1960s in Berkeley, California, at Peet's Coffee and Tea, where one of the founders of Starbucks learned to roast. The regular roast given these days to Peet's Kenyan, for instance, is oily dark, but it has a richness and a grateful sweetness by comparison with the darker so-called Italian or the black French, which inhabits a narrow zone just short of conflagration. To break the crust on a taster's cup of it is to smell tar, licorice, and creosote from a poorly managed woodstove, adding up to an almost mentholated pungency. In the mouth, it is deeply bitter and unpleasant. Does anyone drink it? An extraordinary thing!

Starbucks is no Peet's. And to cup coffee with Dave Olsen and Kevin Knox of the company is to discover a passionate devotion to the coffee bean as well as a fund of knowledge. Certainly, you can discern many fine differences among top coffees as roasted by Starbucks. But the palate changes somewhat; perceptions of spice, for example, seem to increase. Other Seattle roasters, such as SBC Coffee and Caravali, produce somewhat lighter roasts than Starbucks. And not all Western roasters have succumbed to the dark pattern. In the town of Fort Bragg in Mendocino County, California, the good small roaster called Thanksgiving Coffee roasts to a full range of colors.

Significantly, in Seattle the overwhelmingly favorite coffee drink at any time of day is *caffè latte:* a shot of espresso in a cup full of steamed milk topped with foam. (A cappuccino in Italy tastes strongly of espresso under the foam; in America a cappucino is more like an American *caffè latte.*) *Caffè latte* is a well-diluted, usually sweetened drink in which the strong, bitter flavors are very much present but attenuated. Once you grow accustomed to the dark-roast flavors in this approachable form, you may miss them in other milder roasts. That probably explains Seattleites' affection for their *lattes*, although the low acidity of dark roasts may play a part. Seattleites don't favor straight espresso (and certainly not an American-style brew). What many real espresso lovers everywhere prefer is a *ristretto*, a short, black, extra-concentrated cup of espresso made by cutting off the flow of hot water early.

The question remains: Is the color of the roast merely a matter of individual taste? Is there no ideal for each coffee? I believe that there is at least an approximate ideal for each lot of coffee, except that for espresso the beans (lesser ones) might be roasted darker for a different, still-sweet range of tastes. To me, the dominant Seattle style is eccentric, although I've tried to consider it without bias. Starbucks' espresso roast is slightly rasping in the throat. I think the roast for espresso should be ended at about that second crack — roughly the timing that prevails in the northern half of Italy. And for other forms of brewing, taking the example of La Minita, I find the greatest display of aromatics at the lighter end of the range chosen by serious roasters, specifically the style chosen by Green Mountain Coffee Roasters. Admittedly, this is the source closest to me, but I suggest that anyone makes a comparison before concluding that I merely like what I'm used to.

To speak of storing coffee at all is sad, but most people live too far from a roaster to avoid that. Of course, you should buy only whole beans and grind them just before brewing; the goodness in exposed grounds quickly dissipates. And roasted whole beans should be sealed tightly to keep out oxygen and off-flavors and keep in aroma. There are high-tech bags with one-way plastic valves to keep out air yet release carbon dioxide (a powerful degassing occurs in the hours after roasting). I don't disparage them; they are said to work very well for some weeks if the coffee goes into them immediately after roasting. But as a rule freshness is all. Beans for sale anywhere ought to show the date of roasting, and ideally those unprotected by the valves should not be more than three days old. Unfortunately, even most specialty roasters regard this as an impossible standard, but often you can look at dates or ask questions and confine your choices to only the freshest beans.

Some roasters are wary of freezing or even of the chill of the refrigerator. Umberto Bizzarri, an Italian roaster who now works in Seattle, explains that the oils congeal and then prevent the formation of a proper *crema* on a cup of espresso, and that the cold prevents the development of flavor in the beans that occurs after roasting. After asking the opinion of a number of roasters, I conclude that if coffee beans are to be used within a few days of roasting, they ought to be stored at room temperature.

That's fine for professional roasters, who always have fresh beans. For most people, however, it's best to hurry day-old beans home to a tightly sealed glass jar and into the freezer. Room temperature is highly destructive to flavor after a few days, and within ten days the oils on dark-roasted beans begin to turn rancid. Kept frozen, roasted beans are adequately fresh for about two weeks and tolerable for a little longer. Whatever is lost through freezing (perhaps some aromatic high notes) is more than compensated for by all that is saved. Even in 1935, William Ukers wrote that coffee belonged in the refrigerator.

The specialists who have analyzed not only coffee but its making say that water is 98.5 percent of every cup. If your tap water contains a lot of chlorine or another off-flavor, it should be filtered, or bottled water should be used. The most effective brewing temperature is between 195 and 205 degrees Fahrenheit, reached by letting the kettle of boiling water sit off the heat for a minute or two. And the ideal portion of solids to extract from the grounds is about 20 percent. Very soft water extracts too much from the bean, so brewing time should be reduced; hard water extracts too little and counteracts acidity. Too-long brewing muddies the taste and makes coffee bitter. Initially during brewing, more of the aromatic components are extracted, with more of the bitter ones following. When coffee is made by dripping through a filter into an individual cup, the lower strata are the most aromatic; a sip is more pleasant after the coffee has been stirred.

An extraordinary number of coffee-making devices has been invented in the last two centuries, and the brewing method dictates the size of the grind. Coarser grounds suit longer steeping and prevent clogging of the fine holes of some ceramic and metal filters; very fine granules suit the instantaneity of espresso. Some coffee mills are more accurate than others. I use a handsome hand-turned Italian mill, but the inexpensive and miraculously fast electric blade grinders (Krups, Braun, etc.) are excellent. With any blade grinder, it is important to replace a dull blade.

The best way to make coffee depends on what you think good coffee is. It is never weak. But is it clear, or is it murky and rich with the chalky taste of suspended sediment? Is coffee a first-thing-in-the-morning drink with milk, a midmorning or afternoon drink apart from a meal, or a drink with or after dessert? Sediment does add certain flavors and seems to be associated with a chocolaty taste. With different effects, coffee can be made by *infusion*: in the cup, like a professional cupper, or in a Melior-style plunger pot. Or it can be made by the *drip method*: in Chemex and Melitta paper-filter pots and in pots, including the reversible Italian Napoletana, with perforated metal or ceramic filters. Or it can be made by *vacuum*: in Cona brand and other pots, which produce the thinnest, most transparent coffee with the clearest display of aroma. Or it can be made by *pressure*: espresso, a cup of which uses less ground coffee than an

American-style cup. Brewing lasts from as little as fifteen seconds for espresso to two to four minutes for infusion and up to about six minutes for drip. It's better to err by brewing too quickly and too strong rather than too slowly and too weak. Prepare coffee "affectionately" says Claudia Roden in her book *Coffee,* and you can't put it better than that.

The so-called percolator is a miserable boiler of coffee, which drives the delicious aroma into the atmosphere. Its invention is sometimes unfairly attributed to the American-born British loyalist Benjamin Thompson, Count Rumford. But in his monograph *Of the Excellent Qualities of Coffee and the Art of Making It in the Highest Perfection,* he cleverly envisioned holding the liquid at an even temperature by surrounding it with hot water in a special double-jacketed pot, so not even convection currents would circulate the coffee and increase the loss of volatile aromatics from the surface. He roasted his coffee to a "deep cinnamon colour," which I take to mean the color of the unground bark — but that takes us back to roasts.

A paper or cloth filter produces an attractively clear cup, but those filters mute flavor, reduce body, and absorb all the oils. And paper filters contribute a paper taste, some brands more than others. When paper or cloth is replaced by a reusable gold-plated filter, the oils and a portion of fine particles pass into the cup. If you use the old methods of pouring the hot water onto the grounds by hand, first moisten them with a little water. And then after a moment, when they have swollen to form a less permeable layer, add the rest of the water gradually, over no more than eight minutes.

Most of the automatic electric drip machines don't heat water as hot as 195 to 205 degrees Fahrenheit, but they are convenient. And if they do produce really hot water, and if the paper filter is replaced with a gold-plated one (made to fit many brands), then the coffee is very good. Larger quantities are more successful. Avoid using the warming element under the pot.

Aluminum can taint coffee; glass or ceramic pots are best. They must be cleaned with soap and water, since a residue of oils turns into a rancid film. It can be detached by soaking coffee utensils in water and baking soda.

I currently make my coffee in a plunger pot, or I make a single cup with grounds and near-boiling water in a cup and then strain the coffee through a gold-plated filter into a second preheated cup. (I adore espresso but don't make it at home.) The plunger design is French, and the coffee from it is meant to be served in a demitasse. Heavy sediment settles to the bottom of each cup, and the coffee must be brewed strong to be good, I suspect to somehow balance the effect of the sediment. Even after the plunge, the suspended particles keep on brewing and extracting undesirable elements, so the coffee must be drunk promptly. But coffee should always be drunk promptly (possibly excepting coffee held in a vacuum pitcher or thermos). It should never be kept over heat and never reheated. Making coffee and drinking it are essentially one activity; it is a drink of the moment.

One of Luciano De Crescenzo's philosophizing Neapolitans in *Thus Spake Bellavista* remarks, "You must remember, my friend, that coffee is not simply a liquid but something that is, so to speak, halfway between liquid and air; a concoction that, as soon as it touches the palate, is sublimated and instead of going down goes up and up until it enters the brain, where it nestles in a companionable sort of way so that for hours on end a man can be working and thinking, 'What a wonderful cup of coffee I had this morning!'" He elaborates, later in the day: "When a civilized man requires a cup of coffee, it's not because he needs to drink coffee but because he has felt the urge to renew his connection with humanity; he is therefore obliged to interrupt whatever work he happens to be doing, invite one or two colleagues to join him, stroll in the sunshine to his favorite bar, win a minor altercation about who is going to pay, say something complimentary to the girl at the cash register, and exchange a few comments on the sporting scene with the bartender, all without giving the slightest hint about how he likes his coffee, because a proper bartender knows his customers' tastes already. This is a ritual, a religion."

One Seattle roaster and proprietor of two stylish espresso bars remains almost disconnected from the American scene. His approach contradicts the knowledgeable, even cerebral, appreciation that prevails among other fine American roasters. Umberto Bizzarri of Torrefazione Italia started business in Seattle in 1986, having left his home city of Perugia to escape the intense competition in Italy and the partly controlled coffee prices that have put a squeeze on quality. Cheap robustas now form a majority of some Italian blends.

Umberto Bizzarri respects his competition and is grateful to them for introducing Seattle to good coffee. But clearly what they do doesn't interest him, and until I proposed it to him he was unaware of the notion of *terroir* in coffee. What he offers is his palate, expressed through his seven blends (one decaffeinated), which are all he sells and which to him express the range of coffee flavor. He explains simply, "This is my way. I learn from my father," but, "I think I have a different palate from my father." The blends are named for cities — starting with Milano and darkening progressively to Palermo. His favorite, naturally, is Perugia. And his roasts are lighter than those of Starbucks ("It's like burned coffee"), although Palermo comes perilously close. Umberto Bizzarri finds the usual cupping of samples barbaric. When he tastes his beans, he does so after they've been brewed in an espresso machine or a Moka pot.

There may be a danger in analyzing too closely; coffee isn't wine. As the great Fernand Point of the restaurant La Pyramide wrote, "*En cuisine, il faut tout lire, tout voir, tout entendre, tout essayer, tout observer, pour ne retenir en fin de compte qu'assez peu de choses!*" ("In cooking, one must read everything, see everything, hear everything, try everything, observe everything, so as to retain in the end very little!") Only so much conscious appreciation.

Recipes

These few recipes are either instructions for preparations mentioned in the text or examples of the uses of particular ingredients.

LABIATAE: SOME HERBS OF THE MINT FAMILY

Cod with Tomato, Hyssop, and Tarragon

1 small onion, finely chopped
olive oil
½ cup white wine
2 large tomatoes, peeled, seeded, and chopped
1 teaspoon fresh tarragon leaves, coarsely chopped
4 teaspoons fresh hyssop leaves, coarsely chopped
salt and pepper
2 pounds cod, haddock, or pollock, fileted
croutons sautéed in olive oil

In a metal baking dish or in a separate pan, cook the onion in the olive oil over medium heat, without browning, until the onion is translucent. Add the white wine, and boil to reduce the liquid by half. Add the tomatoes, boil for 1 minute, then add the chopped herbs. Season with salt and pepper, and transfer the sauce to a baking dish if it is not already in one.

Wipe the fish with a damp paper towel to pick up any loose scales, and arrange the filet or filets in the baking dish, tucking thin tails under. Drizzle olive oil over the fish and lightly season the upper surface with salt. Bake in a 400° F oven for 6 to 12 minutes, then check the color and texture of the thickest part of the fish with the point of a knife. Remove from the oven as soon as the flesh loses its raw translucence and turns opaque white. Serve immediately strewn with croutons. Serves 4.

Moules à la Marinière

To open mussels as a preliminary to another preparation, cook them as below, adding to the pot several branches of parsley, a bay leaf, and a good pinch of thyme and only optionally including the olive oil or butter, onion or shallot, and garlic. In any case, the precise ingredients of *moules à la marinière* vary. I often prefer olive oil to the butter that is proper to the recipe. If the recipe requires doubling, add only half as much more wine.

> *2 pounds mussels*
> *1 medium onion or large shallot, finely chopped*
> *2 cloves garlic, finely chopped or merely crushed with
>   the flat of a knife*
> *½ cup white wine*
> *1 tablespoon butter*
> *parsley, finely chopped*
> *pepper*

Very fresh mussels do not gape at all, and certainly any mussel should be rejected that does not close soon after it has been knocked about. The shell of an occasional gathered wild mussel is heavy and full of sand. Check by pressing the top shell across the bottom shell, so the two rub across each other slightly; you should feel the strong resistance of the adductor muscle at work. Such gathered mussels should be scrubbed with a brush; farmed mussels can be cleaned by stirring them vigorously with your hands in 2 or 3 changes of water as necessary. Cut off any beards and scrape away any barnacles with a knife.

Cook the onion or shallot and the garlic gently in the wine and butter for a few minutes in a large pot until they are soft. Raise the heat to high, add the mussels, and cover the pot tightly. The mussels usually open in 2 to 3 minutes but may take up to 10 minutes, depending on the quantity and the diameter of the pot. Shake the pot midway or stir the mussels to redistribute them. Remove the pot from the heat as soon as the mussels open. Some will open before others; promptly discard any that do not open at all.

Transfer the mussels to heated soup plates, leaving the liquid behind for a moment to settle. Sprinkle chopped parsley over the mussels, and then pour on the liquid, abandoning the onions and herbs in the bottom of the pot along with the inevitable trace of grit. Have a pepper mill on the table. Serves 4 as a first course, 2 as a main course.

THE ATLANTIC SALMON

Salmon with Cream, Sauternes, and Raisins

If the dish is to be a first course followed by meat and red wine, accompany the salmon with a glass of Sauternes.

> 2½ to 3 pounds salmon, fileted
> white wine
> salt
> ¼ pound mushrooms in thick slices
> ½ teaspoon unsalted butter
> 1 large tomato, peeled, seeded, and chopped
> 2 shallots, finely chopped
> 1 cup heavy cream
> 20 threads saffron
> ½ cup Sauternes

⅓ cup raisins, soaked 1 hour in water and drained
salt and white pepper
1 cucumber
½ teaspoon unsalted butter
salt

Wipe the salmon with a damp paper towel to pick up any loose scales. Find the line of pin bones in the filet or filets and remove them, pinching them with pliers or between thumb and forefinger. Place the salmon skin-side down in an oven dish, pour in white wine to a depth of about ¼ inch, and salt the surface lightly. Cover the dish with kitchen paper, pressing it onto the fish. Bake in a 350° F oven just until a pointed blade reveals that the thickest part is no longer translucent or is almost no longer translucent, according to your taste — about 30 minutes. Remove the dish to a warm spot.

Meanwhile, cook the mushrooms in the butter and a few spoonfuls of water for several minutes over medium-low heat; reserve the mushrooms and their liquid. Cook the tomato briefly over medium heat, so it is nearly purée. Add the shallots and the reserved mushroom liquid, and cook 2 minutes more. Add the cream and the saffron, and cook 5 minutes more. Last, add the Sauternes, reserved mushrooms, and soaked raisins. Season with salt and pepper and remove the sauce from the heat.

Peel the cucumber, halve it, and scrape out the core. Cut the cucumber into roughly 1¼-inch-long julienne sticks. Cook these in ½ teaspoon butter and a few spoonfuls of water for several minutes, until they start to turn translucent. Salt them lightly. Transfer the salmon to a heated platter, pour the sauce over the fish, and arrange the cucumbers around it. Serves 6 as a main course, 10 to 12 as a first course.

Poached, Toasted Country Ham

The length of the standard preliminary soaking is gauged to the dryness of the ham. A younger, moister ham, or a brined ham, is prepared in the same way except that it is soaked for a shorter time or not at all, and various flavorings are put into the cooking liquid. Sawing off the end of the hock allows the ham to fit into the pot, which it may not otherwise do. The piece of hock goes into such things as soup or dried beans, although a smoky hock should first be simmered for 10 minutes in water and the water discarded to rid the hock of crude smoke. A ham is not literally "boiled" as the old recipes say but gently poached. For the first-time ham cook, a thermometer is almost essential to help in regulating the temperature of the water. In general, put the ham to soak the day before cooking, and cook it the day before serving, cooling it overnight. Finish the fat surface on the day the ham is to be served. "Toast," meaning to brown the bread-crumbed surface, is Mary Randolph's word in *The Virginia House-wife*.

> *a whole dry-cured country ham, aged 9 months or more*
> *a ham kettle, 10 gallon stockpot, or another pot measuring*
> *   at least 20 inches in 1 dimension*
> *about 1 cup fine bread crumbs*

Scrub the ham well under warm running water, using a stiff brush to remove mold and superficial matter. Soak the ham in cold water in the cooking pot overnight. Remove the ham, and cut 2 to 3 inches off the hock with a butcher's saw or a clean hacksaw. Discard the soaking water.

Return the ham to the pot and cover with fresh water. Under a loose lid, heat the liquid slowly over a medium flame, until the water steams and sends up steady bubbles, about 2 hours. Promptly lower the heat, so that a bubble rarely if ever rises. (The liquid will be about 180° F.) Poach the ham until with a strong pull you can loosen but not easily free the small bone that reveals itself by the hock — roughly 5 to 7 hours from the time the water reaches poaching temperature. As a rule of thumb: a 15-pound ham is poached in 5½ to 6 hours; add or subtract 20 minutes for each pound above or below 15. Cool the ham overnight in the cooking liquid without moving the pot from the stove.

Place the ham on a large platter or cutting board, and discard the cooking liquid. Remove the discolored surface meat, and cut away the rind to reveal the fat. Trim the fat to an even layer ¼- to ½-inch thick. Cut the aitchbone carefully out of the wide end of the still-warm ham, to permit easy carving. Press the bread crumbs into the fat, and toast well in a 375° F oven, 15 to 20 minutes. Cool the ham for at least ½ hour before carving.

With a well-sharpened knife, preferably a thin slicer with a 12- to 14-inch blade, take several slices off the edge of the ham where the shinbone is nearest the surface — opposite the more rounded, meaty edge. Set the ham on the newly flat area, steady the ham with a carving fork, and remove a wedge of meat near the hock. Starting from the wedge, slice very, very thinly at an angle across the grain. When the meat has been carved from this end, turn the ham end for end. Grasp the shank in a napkin, and carve the meat from the opposite end. Turn the ham over to slice what remains.

ROAST BEEF

Oven-Roasted Standing Ribs of Beef

The entirely optional French style for preparing the roast is to cut away the meat from the tips of the ribs, if they have not been sawn short, so as to show a 1½-inch projection of bone. This highly flavorful meat goes into the stockpot. Salting the meat just before it goes into the oven won't draw out the juices as is sometimes feared, but too much salt will spoil the drippings. Be warned that an electric oven hot enough to brown the roast initially may smoke as the splattering fat hits the hot oven walls. A tight oven will hold this smoke and allow it to settle on the surface of the meat, where it will leave an unpleasant flavor. The only way to avoid this problem is to use a different, presumably gas, oven.

3 to 7 ribs of beef
oil
salt and pepper

Trim the fat, if any has been left by the butcher, to a ¼- to ½-inch layer. If the roast doesn't hold together neatly, tie a loop of string tightly around it between each rib and tie it lengthwise twice. Stand the beef on its ribs in a roasting pan, so the ribs function as a rack, and prevent the bottom of the meat from frying in its fat; if the ribs are cut too short to do the job, place the meat on a metal rack. (In that case, during cooking to compensate for the pan shielding the bottom of the roast from the heat, turn it at least once.) Allow the meat to warm at room temperature for about 2 hours.

Oil the exposed lean, and season the whole with salt and pepper just before placing the beef in the oven. Roast in a preheated 450° F oven for 10 to 15 minutes; then lower the temperature to 350° F and bake, allowing altogether about 15 minutes per pound. But check the temperature of the interior of the roast, normally with a thermometer, well before the period is up. Stop the roasting when the meat is still at least 5 degrees short of the desired temperature of 120° to 125° F for rare, and up to 135° to 140° F for medium. Remove any strings used to tie the meat, transfer the meat to a warm platter, and set in a warm spot. Allow the meat to rest for 20 to 30 minutes before carving. Each 2 pounds of a rib roast will serve about 3 people.

Yorkshire Pudding

1½ cups all-purpose flour
¾ teaspoon salt
1¾ cups milk, at room temperature
3 eggs, at room temperature
drippings from the roasting pan

Time the pudding to go into the oven as soon as the roast comes out, so it will be done just as the roast is served. Whisk together vigorously the flour, salt, milk, and eggs, so as to eliminate all but the tiniest lumps. According to your taste, place 2 tablespoons or much more fat from the roast in a shallow black-steel or copper pan, 10 by 14 inches or an equivalent size. Heat the pan in a 375° F oven to almost smoking, remove the pan, pour in the pudding batter, and return the pan to the oven. Bake until the pudding is puffed and partly brown, 30 to 35 minutes. Bring the hot pan directly to the table. Serves 8 to 12.

EGGS

Crème Renversée au Café

The coffee to go into this custard should be made from freshly roasted beans that are not roasted so dark as to be oily. Afterward, the vanilla bean may be dried and saved for another use. Custard unmolds slightly more easily when cooked in a metal container, such as a tinned charlotte mold. To remove custard from a mold of any material, loosen the edge with the tip of a dull knife and place the serving dish or plate upside down over the mold. Invert the two together. If the custard is reluctant to fall from the mold, hold the two containers securely together and give them a light downward shake to start the movement.

1¼ cups sugar
a flavorless oil or a fresh-tasting nut oil
2¼ cups low-fat milk
¾ vanilla bean, cut crosswise
3 whole eggs plus 3 egg yolks
¾ cup freshly made strong coffee, still warm

Make a caramel of ½ cup of the sugar and 2 tablespoons water, heating them in a small pan over medium-high heat without stirring. After the liquid has colored, there is a brief moment when a wisp of smoke appears but the sugar is not yet burnt. Immediately stir in 2 more tablespoons of water, watching out for dangerous spattering. Stir the caramel until it forms a smooth syrup, and promptly divide it among 8 individual custard cups or molds, tipping each so the caramel lines its lower third to half. Lightly oil the exposed sides.

Heat the milk with the vanilla bean until it comes to a boil. Allow the vanilla to infuse the milk off the heat for 5 minutes, then remove the bean. Mix the whole eggs and egg yolks with the remaining ¾ cup sugar, and stir in the hot milk, gradually at first, and then the coffee. Strain the mixture to remove the chalazae. Pour into the cups or molds, and place them in a large pan filled with very hot water to within half an inch of the tops of the cups. (Metal or glass cups should be set first on a rack or a double layer of paper toweling.) Cover with foil, and poach in a preheated 275° F oven until the custard is set, about 1 hour and 15 minutes. Cool the custard, refrigerating it if necessary, and serve at about 50° F. Unmold only just before serving. Serves 8.

Tahitian Vanilla Ice

¾ cup sugar
3½ cups water
1 Tahitian vanilla bean
½ cup fresh light white wine

Boil the sugar and water together in a small pan until the sugar dissolves; remove the pan from the heat. With a paring knife, split the vanilla bean lengthwise and scrape out the seeds and gel. Stir seeds and gel into the hot sugar syrup. Pour the syrup into another container such as a quart jar, allow it to cool, and add the wine. Cover the mixture and chill it in the refrigerator until it is time to churn the ice. Follow the method for your particular ice cream maker, or make a somewhat coarser ice by freezing the mix in a bowl in the freezer and periodically breaking up the ice crystals with an electric beater. With either method, serve the finished ice, while it is still slightly soft, in cold bowls. Serves 6 to 8.

ENGLISH WALNUTS

Salsa di Noci

Like its obvious kin, basil pesto, this sauce is also Ligurian and was made originally in a mortar. It is served with *tagliatelle* or ravioli (with spinach-stuffed ravioli, use only a little parsley, chopped and stirred in at the end). Preferably, use a flat-leafed Italian variety of parsley. That herb is impossible to measure precisely, but too little in the *salsa di noci* and it requires grated Parmesan at the table; enough parsley and the cheese distracts. The sauce is too rich for a main course of pasta. There are other Ligurian versions of the sauce, as well as similar French sauces for fish, sometimes made with skinned walnuts. *Salsa di noci* can also be served with fish.

1 cup walnuts

1 medium clove garlic

salt

¾ cup parsley leaves, washed and well dried, removed from
*   their stems, and moderately compressed before measuring*

½ cup extra-virgin olive oil

½ cup heavy cream

pepper

Reduce the walnuts to a paste in a food processor. Add the garlic, ¼ teaspoon salt, and the parsley, and again form a paste, scraping down the sides of the bowl of the food processor. Add the oil and process again to form an emulsion. Last, add the cream, processing briefly to combine. Taste and season with salt and pepper. (Heating the sauce will break the emulsion.) Over hot pasta, as a first course, serves 6 to 8.

Sources of Supply

This new, somewhat miscellaneous and personal list of suppliers in North America (plus one in France) goes beyond the limits of the subjects in this book. I've ordered from most of them myself, in some cases repeatedly over a period of years, though never, for instance, from seedhouses specializing in varieties for regions different from my own. With regret, I've left out the important area of American farm cheeses because so many are new and I haven't done enough recent tasting to be sure of my choices.

A Variety of Foodstuffs

Formaggio Kitchen — Ihsan and Valerie Gurdal offer one of the most interesting selections in the United States of high-quality foodstuffs, largely from Western Europe and largely sought out in the places where they are produced. The store has a particular strength in cheese; one of the less obvious strengths is honey. The catalog doesn't reflect the full range or steady changes in what is available.

   244 Huron Avenue
   Cambridge, Massachusetts 02138
   telephone 888.212.3224
   www.formaggiokitchen.com

Zingerman's — This well-known deli and mail-order specialist, founded by Ari Weinzweig and Paul Saginaw, who remain central to the business, covers much of the same ground as the preceding.

But the specific selection is generally different and possibly larger. Beyond the catalog, you can order anything currently stocked in the deli. Zingerman's also excels in cheese.

> 422 Detroit Street
> Ann Arbor, Michigan 48104
> telephone 888.636.8162
> www.zingermans.com

Apples

Each of these nurseries does good work by preserving and propagating old and rare fruit varieties, including some of the most flavorful. Since I haven't planted new fruit trees for years (I'm about to plant a few), I can't vouch from experience for the quality of what is offered. The first listing is a source of apples for tasting, and the last is of a maker of excellent cider vinegar.

Applesource — No trees for sale, but in the fall Tom and Jill Vorbeck ship boxes of apples to taste. That's a boon to anyone trying to decide which varieties to plant. Altogether the Vorbecks offer over one hundred varieties (some in such small quantities that you can learn about them only by calling).

> 1716 Apples Road
> Chapin, Illinois 62628
> telephone 800.588.3854
> www.applesource.com

Big Horse Creek Farm — Ron and Suzanne Joyner, on their farm in the mountains of North Carolina, propagate trees of three hundred antique apple varieties.

> PO Box 70
> Lansing, North Carolina 28643
> telephone 336.384.1134
> www.bighorsecreekfarm.com

Century Farm Orchards — David Vernon, in the northern Piedmont of North Carolina, raises over 450 Southern apple varieties, nearly all of them heirlooms.

> 1614 Rice Road
> Reidsville, North Carolina 27320
> telephone 336.349.5709
> dcvernon@netpath.net

Fedco Trees — The tree division of Fedco, a cooperative known mainly for garden seed (see "Garden Seed"), offers flavorful varieties of fruit, including about four dozen well-described and mostly scarce apples suited to cool and cold climates.

> PO Box 520
> Waterville, Maine 04903
> telephone 207.873.7333
> www.fedcoseeds.com

Greenmantle Nursery — Ram and Marissa Fishman maintain two hundred old apple varieties, including those developed by Albert Etter, whose best-known apple may be the pink-fleshed Pink Pearl and whose best-tasting may be the Wickson.

> 3010 Ettersburg Road
> Garberville, California 95542
> telephone 707.986.7504
> no website

Raintree Nursery — A family-owned nursery offering more than fifty apples chosen for flavor, including a number of heirloom varieties.

> 391 Butts Road
> Morton, Washington 98356
> telephone 360.496.6400
> www.raintreenursery.com

St. Lawrence Nurseries — The fruit trees from the MacKentley family include 150 apple varieties each year out of their collection of more than 200. Many of the apples are old and unusual; all are suited to cold climates.

> 325 State Highway 345
> Potsdam, New York 13676
> telephone 315.265.6739
> www.sln.potsdam.ny.us

Trees of Antiquity — The catalog of this nursery, successor to Sonoma Antique Apple Nursery, lists about 140 antique apples, well-described, out of about 320 heirloom fruits and nuts. Nearly all the apple trees are certified organic.

> 20 Wellsona Road
> Paso Robles, California 93446
> telephone 805.467.2509
> www.treesofantiquity.com

Verger Pierre Gingras — Maker of the best cider vinegar I know, fermented from the juice of four carefully selected late-season apples. The vinegar spends two years in French oak vats and is bottled unfiltered and unpasteurized. The flavor of the regular vinegar is superior to that of the organic or the balsamic-style. Available in some US and Canadian shops and at the orchard.

> 1132 Rue Grande Caroline
> Rougemont, Quebec JOL 1M0 Canada
> telephone 888.469.4954
> www.cidervinegar.com

Beef

Niman Ranch — This well-known source offers conscientiously raised beef from its network of Western ranches. The cattle are slaughtered at eighteen to twenty-four months, considerably older than current mainstream beef, and the Niman meat is dry-aged. (Fresh beef is also available.) Sold at wholesale to markets and restaurants and directly to retail customers. Niman also sells a much smaller quantity of good California lamb in a red-meat as opposed to a pale, young style, and see "Pork."

    1025 East 12th Street
    Oakland, California 94606
    telephone 510.808.0340
    www.nimanranch.com

Coffee

GHH Select — The eight to ten coffees offered by this purist roaster are surely the most discriminating selection in the US. George Howell combines the skills of a longtime professional with the passion of a disinterested connoisseur. He stresses geographic origin, preferring the crop of a single farm in regions where that is available. Apart from the beans for espresso, for which the roast recently was slowly evolving, Howell adheres to a carefully calibrated medium roast that allows the aromatic qualities of the beans to show clearly.

    312 School Street
    Acton, Massachusetts 01720
    telephone 866.444.5282
    www.ghhselect.com

Cornmeal, New England and Southern

Anson Mills — Glenn Roberts, a deeply informed expert on traditional Southern grain, offers stone-ground white and yellow grits from historic varieties of corn. Everything is certified organic; Roberts raises and mills his grain with near-fanatical care and methods. In 2005, his company will begin to sell old-style hominy grits produced using lye from wood ash. Probably they will be the only such grits in commerce.

1922-c Gervais Street
Columbia, South Carolina 29201
telephone 803.467.4122
www.ansonmills.com

Hoppin' John's — Hoppin' John Taylor, an authority on the cooking of the South Carolina Low Country, sells white grits that are stone-ground for him at a mill in north Georgia. The corn is grown from traditional varieties by local Georgia farmers and dried in the field in the old way.

PO Box 12775
Charleston, South Carolina 29412
telephone 800.828.4412
www.hoppinjohns.com

Morgan's Mills — Rhode Island white flint corn, the traditional kind grown around the Narragansett Bay, is stone-ground in Maine by Richard Morgan, a Rhode Island native. The cornmeal is ideal for New England cornbread and jonnycakes.

168 Payson Road
Union, Maine 04862
telephone 207.785.4900
morgan@midcoast.com

Earthenware

Henderson's Redware — Kenneth Henderson produces, by hand, traditional American earthenware (redware) cooking pots and other containers: bean pots, colanders, bowls, preserve jars, lard pots, pipkins.

2115 Union Street
Bangor, Maine 04401
telephone 866.376.4475
www.hendersonsredware.com

Garden Seed and Potatoes

During the 1980s, a low point for home vegetable gardeners, the number of seedhouses was shrinking, old vegetable varieties were being abandoned and lost, and few new vegetable varieties of any kind were being introduced that had been bred expressly for home gardens. The seed business was focused on the big money: varieties with qualities suited to large-scale commercial production. Yet in the last ten years, public attention has returned to old-fashioned flavorful varieties. New businesses have appeared, selling seed of heirloom vegetables, and steadily uncovering more of them. (Still, the number of varieties of a few commonplace items has been slow to rebound: beets, cabbage, turnips, onions.) The following are just some of the seedhouses that defend flavor and diversity in vegetables.

Baker Creek Heirloom Seeds — Founded in 1998 by Jere Gettle, who was then only eighteen. He now offers eight hundred vegetable varieties, including a number of heirlooms from Southeast Asia. Descriptions in many cases are limited.

> 2278 Baker Creek Road
> Mansfield, Missouri 65704
> telephone 417.924.8917
> www.rareseeds.com

Fedco Seeds — The corporate-sounding name stands for the very non-corporate "Federation of cooperatives," and the black-and-white catalog has character. It lists many organic seeds and heirloom varieties, such as Costata Romanesca zucchini (almost the only kind to grow for flavor) and historic northern New England flint corns inherited from the Native American tribes who first lived in the region. Low prices. (For the separate catalog devoted to trees, see "Apples.")

> PO Box 520
> Waterville, Maine 04903
> telephone 207.873.7333
> www.fedcoseeds.com

High Mowing Seeds — Regionally adapted, open-pollinated varieties, including many heirlooms. All are certified organic.

    813 Brook Road
    Wolcott, Vermont 05680
    telephone 802.888.1800
    www.highmowingseeds.com

Native Seeds/SEARCH — This nonprofit sells seeds of traditional crops of the Native American tribes of the southwestern US and northwestern Mexico, especially corn, beans, and squash. These old varieties are suited to desert conditions.

    526 North Fourth Avenue
    Tucson, Arizona 85705
    telephone 520.622.5561
    www.nativeseeds.org

Ronniger's — The Ronniger family farm produces a large selection of potato varieties for planting (and at wholesale for eating), all certified organic.

    HCR 62, Box 332A
    Moyie Springs, Idaho 83845
    telephone 208.267.7938
    www.ronnigers.com

Salt Spring Seeds — Many unique varieties; all seed is open-pollinated and organically grown, and — almost unheard of — this seller grows all its own seed.

    Box 444, Ganges PO
    Salt Spring Island, BC v8k 2w1 Canada
    telephone 250.537.5269
    www.saltspringseeds.com

Seed Savers Exchange — The catalog of this nonprofit has the widest commercial selection I know of heirloom vegetable varieties. Some seed is organic. Profits go toward maintaining the SSE's collection of twenty-four thousand rare varieties of vegetables.

> 3076 North Winn Road
> Decorah, Iowa 52101
> telephone 563.382.5990
> www.seedsavers.org

Southern Exposure Seed Exchange — Seed of open-pollinated varieties (with half a dozen exceptions), most of them traditional. All are suited to the central Atlantic region, and much of the seed is organic. A for-profit business run with a nonprofit mentality.

> PO Box 460
> Mineral, Virginia 23117
> telephone 540.894.9480
> www.southernexposure.com

Territorial Seed Company — The selection of varieties emphasizes flavor. Some are open-pollinated heirlooms; some are modern hybrids. A portion of the seed is organic, and the company operates forty-four acres of certified organic trial grounds.

> PO Box 158
> Cottage Grove, Oregon 97424
> telephone 541.942.9547
> www.territorial-seed.com

Wood Prairie Farm — Jim and Megan Gerritsen offer a modest-sized selection of well-grown potatoes, both seed potatoes and eating potatoes, all certified organic.

> 49 Kinney Road
> Bridgewater, Maine 04735
> telephone 800.829.9765
> www.woodprairie.com

Ham, Aged Southern Country, and Country Bacon

S. Wallace Edwards and Son — The ham to buy is the Wigwam, cured with salt and a little sodium nitrate, then hickory smoked, pepper-coated, and aged for ten to twelve months. After Christmas, the aged hams may be sold out for a time. The bacon, while good, comes sealed in plastic and is milder than traditional country bacon. The largest amount, a half slab, comes with the rind on; smaller amounts have the rind removed and are sliced.

    PO Box 25
    Surry, Virginia 23883
    telephone 800.222.4267
    www.virginiatraditions.com

R.M. Felts Packing Co. — Producer of my longtime favorite bacon, cured with only salt, then pepper-coated and smoked with damp oak sawdust. Jowls are similarly cured and also good. Either one is shipped properly wrapped in greaseproof paper, not in plastic. You can order the bacon sliced, but slab bacon holds its flavor much better. All the bacon comes, as it should, with the rind on, and you can still get a "rib side," which is a whole slab with the ribs in. I have never tried the dry-cured hams, which are sold young, after only ninety days.

    PO Box 199
    Ivor, Virginia 23866
    telephone 757.859.6131
    no website

Gatton Farms (Father's Country Hams) — The Gatton family ham cure contains salt, sugar, sodium nitrate, and sodium nitrite. The hams are smoked with green hickory and aged nine to twelve months, and in some cases longer. The bacon, from which the rind has been removed, is a little too smoky for my taste. You can buy it in slabs; smaller amounts are sliced and sealed in plastic.

PO Box 99
Bremen, Kentucky 42325
telephone 877.525.4267
www.fatherscountryhams.com

Colonel Bill Newsom — This ham is cured with only salt, no nitrate or nitrite; a little brown sugar is added. The ham is smoked over green hickory and then aged hock downward, on the theory that makes a plumper, moister ham, for a minimum of ten months. Nancy Mahaffey, daughter of the late Colonel Bill, says the business was started in 1917 but that the family has been curing hams in Kentucky by the same method since 1798. (Newsom's also sells excellent traditional sorghum syrup, milled not far away by Amish using horse power.) No bacon.

Newsom's Old Mill Store
208 East Main Street
Princeton, Kentucky 42445
telephone 270.365.2482
www.newsomscountryham.com

Herbs: Oregano and Sage

Kalustyan's — For bags of whole branches of dried oregano and sage from Greece, both of which I believe are gathered in the wild (the same herbs are sold at many Greek markets).

123 Lexington Avenue
New York, New York 10016
telephone 212.685.3451
www.kalustyans.com

Hickory Nuts, Shagbark

Wisconsin Wild Fruits — Jennifer De Bolt gathers the hard-shelled shagbark hickory nuts from untended trees and then shells them, which is no small task. That makes the price for shagbark hickory nuts higher than for other shelled nuts, but shagbark hickory nuts are one of the best kinds of all. Before you eat them, you must toast them: spread them on a baking sheet and place them in a 250 degree F oven for three to fifteen minutes, according to your taste.

PO Box 1263
Madison, Wisconsin 53703
telephone (home) 608.239.9040
wisconsinwildfruits@yahoo.com

Lamb

Jamison Farm — John and Sukey Jamison produce lamb in a tender pale style that recalls milk-fed. They buy just-weaned lambs from surrounding farms and raise them on their 160 acres of intensively managed pasture. The lambs are finished on grass, not grain, and carefully slaughtered at four to six months. Normally the meat is shipped frozen to retail customers — be sure to ask for fresh.

171 Jamison Lane
Latrobe, Pennsylvania 15650
telephone 800.237.5262
www.jamisonfarm.com

Maple Syrup

Gadapee Family Sugarhouse — Each sugarbush, and even each day, produces sap that gives maple syrup with different flavor, from subtle to distinct. The way to pay a moderate price is to buy a gallon directly from a producer. Once the container has been opened, occasionally yeast forms on the surface of the syrup inside and if left long enough will affect the taste. To discourage that possibility, keep the container refrigerated and never, after you pour syrup out, pour any back in. This syrup is made by the Gadapee family, especially Keith and his father Larry, using a wood-fired evaporator. Sugar-making in this area typically runs from early March into April; by late winter, a producer has often run out of syrup.

718 Calkins Camp Road
Danville, Vermont 05828
telephone 802.684.3323
gadmaple@together.net

Mustard, English

Belgravia Imports — The mustards of the Tracklement Company, Ltd., known as Wiltshire Tracklements at the time of the first edition of this book, are brought from the UK to the US by Belgravia Imports. Many European mustards are made differently for the US market, and they tend to be old by the time they reach US retail shelves, so the taste has little in common with what is enjoyed in the home country. Tracklements Company mustards, however, are made the same for everyone, and they arrive in the US in a fresher state than most European mustards do. My favorite is the one called Black Mustard, made with black pepper. Ordering directly from Belgravia, the main importer, further increases the likelihood that you will taste the mustard at its prime. The good qualities of any mustard, whether or not the jar has yet been opened, are best preserved in the refrigerator.

1430 East Main Road
Portsmouth, Rhode Island 02871
telephone 800.848.1127
belgravia@belgraviaimports.com

Pecans, Wild

Circle's Pecans — Tom and Linda Circle cultivate 120 acres of pecan trees. As on many farms in their region, some of the trees are wild in origin and others are "improved" varieties. I'm one of those who believe the wild pecans, which are smaller and have thicker shells, are more flavorful. It's best to buy them fresh just after the harvest, which begins in late October and runs into December. Then you can seal the nuts tightly in glass jars and freeze them, which is the best way to store any nuts. When ordering from the Circles, be sure to specify "native" nuts, unless you want to make a comparison.

> 2499 US Highway 400
> McCune, Kansas 66753
> telephone (business) 620.632.4382
> telephone (home) 620.632.4236
> www.circlespecans.com

Plum Pudding

Mother Sperry's Plum Pudding — The real thing made properly by Winnie Sperry using beef suet, since 1980.

> 1416 East Aloha Street
> Seattle, Washington 98112
> telephone (home office) 206.329.8631
> no website

Pork

Niman Ranch — Unlike mainstream pork, Niman Ranch pork is well-marbled and humanely raised. Niman pork sales have steadily grown, which means more decent family farms are able to stay in business. The meat is sold at wholesale to markets and restaurants as well as directly to retail customers. (See also "Beef.")

> 1025 East 12th Street
> Oakland, California 94606
> telephone 510.808.0340
> www.nimanranch.com

Salmon, Fresh and Smoked

10th and M Seafoods — Supplier of fresh wild Alaska salmon (king, sockeye, coho, pink, chum) in season. The website's chart of the seasons provides a rough guide; call to learn what is available that day.

> 1020 M Street
> Anchorage, Alaska 99501
> telephone 800.770.2722
> www.10thandmseafoods.com

Tustumena Smokehouse — Fred West's delicious "old-style" hot-smoked wild Alaska salmon is traditional, except that less salt is used than in the days before refrigeration. In the course of hot-smoking, the salmon is cooked and thus very different from familiar, cold-smoked salmon. Freshly caught (not previously frozen) smoked fish are available from roughly June through July, the species depending on what is running at the time.

> 30022 Kimberly Street
> Soldotna, Alaska 99669
> telephone 907.260.3401
> www.tustumenasmokehouse.com

Salt

The most economical way to buy gray sea salt that I've found is in five-kilo or larger sacks from a natural foods store. If a store doesn't stock the salt, it may be willing to place a special order. I recently paid about $2.25 per pound.

Sauerkraut

Wellspring Farm — Les Snow slices and ferments his farm's organic cabbage, adding a minimum of gray Breton sea salt and nothing else. (He took over the sauerkraut part of Hill Farm, described in this book.) The outstanding sauerkraut, sold raw as it should be, is sold in some stores in the Northeast, and Snow ships directly to individual customers.

190 Lafiria Place
Marshfield, Vermont 05658
telephone 802.426.3890
www.wellspringfarmvt.com

Sorghum Syrup

Townsend's Sorghum Mill — Sorghum syrup, with its tang and mild molasses flavor, was formerly a main sweetening in much of the South, as maple sugar was in the North. The Townsend family raises the sorghum cane and makes the syrup.

11620 Main Street
Jeffersonville, Kentucky 40337
telephone (home) 859.498.4142
no website

Spices

Penzeys Spices — This ever-expanding purveyor, which recently had seventeen shops, offers a wide variety of high-quality spices, including Tellicherry extra-bold black pepper and Vietnamese and Chinese cassia. The ground spices, such as ginger, are fresh and potent. Herbs are also good though less special than the spices.

PO Box 924
Brookfield, Wisconsin 53008
telephone 800.741.7787
www.penzeys.com

Tea

Tea offers one of the greatest, perhaps the greatest, experience of taste — subtle, extremely varied and complex. It probably goes without saying that only whole-leaf teas are of interest, never tea in bags.

Imperial Tea Court — Roy and Grace Fong's traditional teahouse, built by craftsmen from China, is a source of outstanding Chinese teas.

> 1411 Powell Street
> San Francisco, California 94133
> telephone 800.567.5898
> www.imperialtea.com

In Pursuit of Tea — Sebastian Beckwith, Frank Kwei, and Alexander Scott are passionate tea lovers; they offer excellent teas from China as well as a few from Darjeeling in India and elsewhere.

> 224 Roebling Street
> Brooklyn, New York 11211
> telephone 866.878.3832
> www.inpursuitoftea.com

Kyela Teas — The one-person business of my friend Kevin Gascoyne is, I believe, the world's finest source of Darjeeling, just ten to twenty top teas each year, most of them otherwise unavailable in North America. Gascoyne visits Darjeeling annually to taste. He aims to run out before the first new teas of the year arrive in early June, so his teas are fresh, an important point with Darjeeling and all but a few exceptional teas.

> 4057 Avenue de l'Esplanade
> Montreal, Quebec H2W 1S9 Canada
> no telephone
> www.kyelateas.com

La Maison des Trois Thés — This unique teahouse located near the Place Monge in Paris is probably the finest source anywhere, including China, of tea from China, and it is an exceptional place to taste. To gain an idea of how broad and deep the selection is, you may have to ask specific, informed questions. There are great blue-greens (oolongs) from Taiwan, birthplace of Madame Tseng, one of the world's few tea masters, who is responsible for La Maison des Trois Thés.

> 33 Rue Gracieuse
> 75005 Paris France
> telephone 33.01.4336.9384
> info@maisondestroisthes.com

Wild Rice

Native Harvest (White Earth Land Recovery Project) — The wild rice (*Zizania palustris*, to use the preferred botanical name) sold by the Ojibway of the White Earth Reservation is collected by hand, the gatherers working from canoes, as required by Minnesota law. Not to be confused with the black cultivated version of the grain, the truly wild is olive green, brown, and tan in color, and it tastes much, much better.

> 33287 County Highway 34
> Ogema, Minnesota 56569
> telephone 888.779.3577
> www.welrp.org

Bibliography

This bibliography, from the original edition, was chosen primarily to suggest further reading and some useful cookbooks rather than to serve as a list of sources.

General Books and Cookbooks

David, Elizabeth. *Elizabeth David Classics: A Book of Mediterranean Food, French Country Cooking, Summer Cooking.* New York: Alfred A. Knopf, 1980.

——. *French Provincial Cooking.* New York: Penguin, 1970.

——. *Italian Food.* New York: Penguin, 1977.

——. *An Omelette and a Glass of Wine.* New York: Viking, 1985.

Davidson, Alan. *A Kipper with My Tea.* London: Macmillan, 1988; San Francisco: North Point Press, 1990.

The Good Cook. Series. Alexandria, Va.: Time-Life, 1979–83.

Gray, Patience. *Honey from a Weed.* New York: Harper & Row, 1987.

Hartley, Dorothy. *Food in England.* London: Macdonald & Co., 1954.

——. *Lost Country Life.* New York: Pantheon Books, 1979.

Kamman, Madeleine. *When French Women Cook.* New York: Atheneum, 1976.

Liebling, A.J. *Between Meals: An Appetite for Paris.* San Francisco: Simon & Schuster, 1962.

Martha Washington's Booke of Cookery. Transcribed and annotated by Karen Hess. New York: Columbia University Press, 1981.

McGee, Harold. *On Food and Cooking.* New York: Charles Scribner's Sons, 1984.

Olney, Richard. *The French Menu Cookbook*. Rev. ed. Boston: David Godine, 1985.

———. *Simple French Food*. New York: Atheneum, 1974.

Pépin, Jacques. *The Art of Cooking*. 2 vols. New York: Alfred A. Knopf, 1987–88.

Randolph, Mary. *The Virginia House-wife*. Washington, D.C.: 1924. Facsimile edition with historical notes and commentaries by Karen Hess. Columbia: University of South Carolina Press, 1984.

Saint-Ange, E. *La Cuisine de Madame Saint-Ange*. Paris: Librairie Larousse, 1982.

White, Florence, ed. *Good Things in England*. London: Jonathan Cape, 1951.

Books and Articles on Specific Subjects

TOMATOES, CARROTS, AND MUSTARD

Banga, O. *Main Types of the Western Carotene Carrot and Their Origin*. Wageningen, Netherlands: Institute for Horticultural Plant Breeding, 1963.

Boswell, Victor R. "Improvement and Genetics of Tomatoes, Peppers, and Eggplant," *Yearbook of Agriculture*. Washington, D.C.: Government Printing Office, 1937.

Coe, Sophie. *America's First Cuisines*. Austin, Tex.: University of Texas, 1994.

———. "Aztec Cuisine, Part II," *Petits Propos Culinaires* 20, July 1985.

Decloquement, Françoise. *Moutardes et moutardiers*. Paris: Bréa Editions, 1983.

Leighton, Ann. *American Gardens in the Eighteenth Century*. Boston: Houghton Mifflin, 1976.

———. *Early American Gardens*. Boston: Houghton Mifflin, 1970.

Man, Rosamond, and Robin Weir. *The Compleat Mustard*. London: Constable and Co., 1988.

Smith, Andrew F. *The Tomato in America*. Columbia, S.C.: University of South Carolina, 1994.

MUSSELS AND SALMON

Berrill, Michael, and Deborah Berrill. *A Sierra Club Naturalists' Guide to the North Atlantic Coast*. San Francisco: Sierra Club Books, 1981.

Brown, Bruce. *Mountain in the Clouds: A Search for the Wild Salmon*. New York: Simon & Schuster, 1982.

Davidson, Alan. Mediterranean Seafood. 2d ed. London: Allen Lane, 1981.

——. North Atlantic Seafood. New York: Viking, 1980.

Dunfield, R.W. The Atlantic Salmon in the History of North America. Ottawa: Department of Fisheries and Oceans, 1985.

Netboy, Anthony. The Atlantic Salmon: A Vanishing Species? Boston: Houghton Mifflin, 1968.

Ricketts, Edward F., Jack Calvin, and Joel W. Hedgpeth. Between Pacific Tides. 5th ed. Stanford, Calif.: Stanford University Press, 1985.

Schneider, Elizabeth. "Mussel-bound in Maine: The Art of the State," The Journal of Gastronomy. Vol. 4, no. 4, 1989.

Williamson, Henry. Salar the Salmon. London: Faber & Faber, 1935; Boston: David Godine, 1990.

SALT AND BLACK PEPPER

David, Elizabeth. Spices, Salt, and Aromatics in the English Kitchen. New York: Penguin, 1975.

Disney, A.R. Twilight of the Pepper Empire. Cambridge, Mass.: Harvard University Press, 1978.

Eskew, Garnett Laidlaw. Salt, the Fifth Element. Chicago: J.G. Ferguson, 1948.

Hicks, Alexandra. "Red Peppercorns — What They Really Are," Petits Propos Culinaires 10, March 1982.

Hyman, Philip, and Mary Hyman. "Long Pepper: A Short History," Petits Propos Culinaires 6, October 1980. (See also PPC 12, correspondents' notes on long pepper and pink peppercorns.)

Intersalt Cooperative Research Group. "Intersalt: An international study of electrolyte excretion and blood pressure. Result for 24 hour urinary sodium and potassium excretion," British Medical Journal, vol. 297, pp. 319–28, 1988.

Miller, J. Inness. Spice Trade of the Roman Empire. London: Oxford University Press, 1969.

Moore, Thomas J. "With a grain of salt: Have medical researchers misled the American public about the dangers of dietary sodium?" Eating Well, March–April 1991.

Sass, Lorna. "Religion, Medicine, Politics, and Spices." *The Journal of Gastronomy*. Vol. 4, no. 4, 1989.

Swale, J.D. "Salt saga continued: Salt has only small importance in hypertension," *British Medical Journal*. Vol. 297, pp. 307–308, 1988.

HAM

Jacobs, Jay. "The Art of Prosciutto," *Gourmet*, January 1985.

Lowery, Deborah G. "Country Ham: The Flavor of Tradition," *Southern Living*, October 1986.

EGGS AND CREAM

Androuët, Pierre. *Guide du fromage.* English ed., rev. Nuffield, Oxfordshire: Aidan Ellis, 1983.

Dolnick, Edward. "Does It Matter What We Eat?" *La Varenne Newsletter*, Winter 1991.

———. *"Le paradoxe français:* How do the French eat all that rich food and skip the heart disease?" *In Health*, May–June 1990.

Houghton, Frederick L. *Holstein-Friesian Cattle: A History of the Breed and Its Development in America.* Brattleboro, Vt.: Press of the Holstein-Friesian Register, 1897.

Le Jaouen, Jean-Claude. *La Fabrication du fromage de chèvre fermier.* Paris: ITOVIC, 1982.

Murphy, Bill. *Greener Pastures on Your Side of the Fence.* Colchester, Vt.: Arriba Publishing, 1987.

Nelson, John A., and G. Malcolm Trout. *Judging Dairy Products.* 4th ed. Milwaukee: Olsen Publishing, 1965.

Rance, Patrick. *The French Cheese Book.* London: Macmillan, 1989.

———. *The Great British Cheese Book.* London: Macmillan, 1988.

Robinson, John H. *Principles and Practice of Poultry Culture.* Boston: Ginn and Co., 1912.

Smith, Page, and Charles Daniel. *The Chicken Book.* Boston: Little, Brown & Co., 1975.

Stacey, Michelle. "Reinventing the Egg," *The New Yorker*, October 1, 1990.

Walstra, Pieter, and Robert Jenness. *Dairy Chemistry and Physics.* New York: John Wiley & Sons, 1984.

Weir, Harrison, et al. *The Poultry Book.* New York: Doubleday, Page and Co., 1904.

APPLES

Beach, S.A. *The Apples of New York.* 2 vols. Albany, N.Y.: J.B. Lyon, 1905.

Bunyard, Edward. *The Anatomy of Dessert.* New York: E.P. Dutton, 1934.

———. *Handbook of Hardy Fruits: Apples and Pears.* London: John Murray, 1925.

Carlson, R.F., et al. *North American Apples: Varieties, Rootstocks, and Outlook.* East Lansing: Michigan State University Press, 1970.

Coxe, William. *A View of the Cultivation of Fruit Trees, etc.* Philadelphia: M. Carery and Son, 1817.

Hedrick, U.P. *Cyclopedia of Hardy Fruits.* 2d ed. New York: Macmillan, 1938.

———. *A History of Horticulture in America.* New York: Oxford University Press, 1950.

Hogg, Robert. *The Fruit Manual.* London: Journal of Horticulture, 1875. (See also other editions.)

Jansen, H.F. "Taste Evaluation of Apples from an Ontario Fruit Garden," *Fruit Varieties and Horticultural Digest,* Vol. 26, no. 4, 1972.

Morgan, Joan. "In Praise of Older Apples," *Petits Propos Culinaires* 20, July 1985.

Nitschke, Robert A. "Apples for Dessert — A Second Look, Parts I and II," *Fruit Varieties and Horticultural Digest.* Vol. 19, nos. 3 and 4, 1965.

———. Catalog (no date) and various annual price lists of Southmeadow Fruit Gardens, Lakeside, Mich.

Roach, F.A. *Cultivated Fruits of Britain.* New York: Basil Blackwell, 1985.

Shand, P. Morton. "Older Kinds of Apples," *Journal of the Royal Horticultural Society,* 1949.

Smith, M.W.G. *National Apple Register of the United Kingdom.* London: Ministry of Agriculture, Fisheries and Food, 1971.

Taylor, H.V. "Apples," *The Orchard and Fruit Garden.* Edited by Edward Hyams and A.A. Jackson. London: Longmans, Green & Co., 1961.

Way, Roger. "My Favorite Dessert Apples," *Fruit Varieties and Horticultural Digest.* January 1966, pp. 18–19.

Westwood, Melvin N. *Temperate-Zone Pomology*. Rev. ed. Portland, Ore.:
    Timber Press, 1988.

VANILLA

Correll, D.S. "Vanilla — Its botany, history, cultivation and economic import,"
    Economic Botany. Vol. 7, 1953, pp. 291–358.
Land, Leslie. "Plain Vanilla," *The Journal of Gastronomy*. Vol. 2, no. 4, 1986.
Matchat, Cecile Hulse. "Vanilla — The Orchid of Commerce," *Orchid Review*,
    February 1934.
Purseglove, J.W., et al. *Spices*. New York: Longmans, 1980.
Rain, Patricia. *Vanilla Cookbook*. Berkeley, Calif.: Celestial Arts, 1986.
Riley, K.A., and D.H. Klein. "Fundamental Principles of Vanilla/Vanilla
    Extract Processing and Methods of Detecting Adulteration in Vanilla
    Extracts," *Food Technology*, October 1989.
Rolfe, R. Allen. "Vanillas of Commerce," *Kew Bulletin*. Vol. 4, 1895.

COFFEE

Clarke, R.J., and R. Macrae, eds. *Coffee*. Vol. 1, *Chemistry*. New York:
    Elsevier Applied Science Publishers, 1985.
Naval Intelligence Division [G.B.]. *Western Arabia and the Red Sea*.
    Oxford [?]: 1946.
Hattox, Ralph S. *Coffee and Coffeehouses*. Seattle: University of Washington
    Press, 1985.
Jobin, Philippe. *The Coffees Produced Throughout the World*. Le Havre: P. Jobin
    et Cie., 1982.
Kummer, Corby. "Before the First Sip," *Atlantic Monthly*, May 1990.
———. "Espresso at Home," *Atlantic Monthly*, November 1990.
———. "Is Coffee Harmful?" *Atlantic Monthly*, July 1990.
———. "Untroubled Brewing," *Atlantic Monthly*, June 1990.
Lingle, Ted. *The Basics of Cupping Coffee*. Washington, D.C.: Coffee
    Development Group, 1986.
Lingle, Ted. *The Coffee Cuppers' Handbook*. Washington, D.C.: Coffee
    Development Group, 1986.

Sivetz, Michael, and Norman W. Desrosier. *Coffee Technology*. Westport, Conn.: AVI Publishing, 1979.

Thompson, Benjamin [Count Rumford]. *Collected Works of Count Rumford*. Vol. 5. Cambridge, Mass.: Belknap Press of Harvard University Press, 1970.

——. *Of the Excellent Qualities of Coffee and the Art of Making It in the Highest Perfection*. London: 1812.

Ukers, William H. *All About Coffee*. 2d ed. New York: The Tea and Coffee Trade Journal Company, 1935.

PERIODICALS ABOUT FOOD

The Art of Eating
PO Box 242
Peacham, Vermont 05862
($39 per year, four issues)

Food History News
1061 Main Road
Islesboro, Maine 04848
www.foodhistorynews.com
($22 per year, four issues)

Petits Propos Culinaires
Allaleigh House
Blackawton, Totnes
Devon TQ9 7DL
United Kingdom
www.prospectbooks.co.uk
($28.50 per year, three issues, checks made payable to PPC North America)

Simple Cooking
PO Box 778
Northampton, Massachusetts 01061
www.outlawcook.com
($25 per year, five issues)

Index

Bay leaves (cont.)
    to support other seasonings, 96
    toxicity of, 94
    Turkish, 96
Bay of Fundy, 51–56
Beach, S.A., 159
Beeton, Mrs. Isabella, 94, 132
Bell peppers, 62
Beranbaum, Rose Levy, 151
Beverley, Robert, 82
Bizzarri, Umberto, 243, 247
Bowman, Sam, 56
Bridges, Bill, 137
Brillat-Savarin, 122, 132, 141, 228
Buist, Robert, 8–9
Bunyard, Edward, 168–69
Burr, Fearing, Jr., 9
Butter, 185
Butterworks Farm, 193–96

Cake Bible, The (Beranbaum), 151
Calvert, Kit, 189
Capsicums, 62
Caravali Coffees, 221, 236, 241
Carrots, sweet orange, 99–111
    balancing effect on other flavors, 109
    color of, 100–01
    cooking of, 108–09
    described, 102–03
    flavor of, 102–07
    growing conditions for, 107
    history of, 99–102
    quality of, 108
    sugar in, 104–07
    varieties of, 110–11
Cheeses, 189
Child, Julia, 93, 94
Chili peppers, 61, 62
Chocolate, 151, 200
Clements, Mrs., 117, 124
Coca-Cola, 201
Coffee, 221–47
    acidity of, 222–23

arabica, 227, 228, 230, 232–38
bitterness of, 224
blended, 237–38
Blue Mountain, 237
brewing of, 243–46
caffeine in, 222, 228–29
caffè latte, 241–42
Catimor, 232
decaffeinated, 228–29
defects in, 231, 234
espresso, 240–41
flavored, 229
flavor of, 223–24
flavor prototypes, 232–38
freshness of, 242–43
growers of, 229–38
health and, 228
milling of, 230–31
Mocha, 233, 234–35
roasting of, 226, 238–42
robusta, 227–28
sampling of, by tasters, 221–27
in Seattle, 240–42, 243, 247
specialty roasters, 221–29
storing of, 242–43
supermarket, 226, 227–28
trees, 229–30
variability of, 227
Yergacheffe, 232–33
Coffee (Roden), 245
Coffee Connection, 221, 224
Coffee Cuppers' Handbook,
    The (Lingle), 224
Coffeehouses, 228, 233–34
Colman, Jeremiah, 118, 124
Colman's mustard, 115–16, 118–19
Columbus, Christopher, 62
Compleat Mustard, The
    (Man and Weir), 126
Corn, 107
Cortés, 200
Costante, Joe, 162
Country Farm, The, 8

porr*The Artful Eater* is set in Abode Jenson, drawn by
Robert Slimbach and issued in 1996.
The design of the roman typeface is based on a font cut
in Venice in 1469 by the French typographer
Nicolas Jenson, and the italic is based on Arrighi,
drawn in 1925 by the American Frederic Warde (from
the work of Ludovico degli Arrighi in the 1520s).

Flourishes and decorative elements are in
ITC Golden Cockerel, drawn by Phill Grimshaw
and based on Eric Gill's designs for
Gold Cockerel Press in 1929.

Designed by Keith Chamberlin for FLEK, Inc.

Printed and bound at Vail-Ballou Press,
Binghamton, New York.